JOHN EBNEZAR CBS | Handbooks in
Orthopedics and Fractures

SERIES

Orthopedic Disease

Disorders of Joints

John Ebnezar

- Holder of the **Guinness Book of World Records** for the most number of books written by an individual in a single year.
- Listed in the **India Book of Records** for the most number of books written by an individual.
- Recipient of the highest civilian awards of Karnataka, the **Rajyotsava Award 2010** and the **Kempegowda Award 2011**.
- Recipient of the **Best Citizen of India Award** by the International Publishing house.
- Former Vice-President, the Indian Orthopaedic Association
- President, Neuro-Spinal Surgeons Association of India (Karnataka)
- CEO, Parimala Health Care Services, A ISO 9001:2008 Hospital, Bilekahalli, Bannerghatta Road, Bangalore
- Ebnezar Orthopedic Center, Bilekahalli, Bannerghatta Road, Bangalore
- Dr John's Orthopedic Clinic, near Reliance Mart, Arakere, BG Road, Bangalore
- Chairman, the Physically Handicapped and Paraplegic Charitable Trust of Karnataka®
- Founder President, Geriatric Orthopedic Society
- Founder President, Orthopedic Authors Association and All India Medical Authors Association
- Chairman, Karnataka Orthopedic Academy®
- President, Bangalore Holistic Academy
- Chairman, Rakesh Cultural Academy
- President, Vaidya Kala Ranga, Bangalore
- Secretary, SK Educational Society®
- Former Senior Specialist, Victoria Hospital, Bangalore Medical College, Bangalore
- Former Assistant Professor in Orthopedics, Devaraj Urs Medical College, Kolar, Karnataka
- Postgraduate teacher, Bangalore Baptist Hospital, Airport Road, Bangalore

John Ebnezar CBS | Handbooks in
Orthopedics and Fractures

SERIES

Orthopedic Disease

Disorders of Joints

John Ebnezar

MBBS, D'Ortho, DNB (Ortho), MNAMS (Ortho), PhD (Yoga)
Sports Medicine (Australia), INOR Fellow (UK), DAc, DMT

Consulting Orthopedic and Spine Surgeon
Holistic Orthopedic Expert, and Sports Specialist
Bangalore

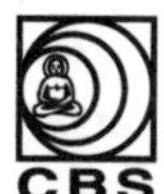

CBS Publishers & Distributors Pvt Ltd

New Delhi • Bengaluru • Pune • Kochi • Chennai

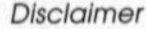

Disclaimer
Science and technology are constantly changing fields. New research and experience broaden the scope of information and knowledge. The author has tried his best in giving information available to him while preparing the material for this book. Although, all efforts have been made to ensure optimum accuracy of the material, yet it is quite possible some errors might have been left uncorrected. The publisher, printer and author will not be held responsible for any inadvertent errors or inaccuracies.

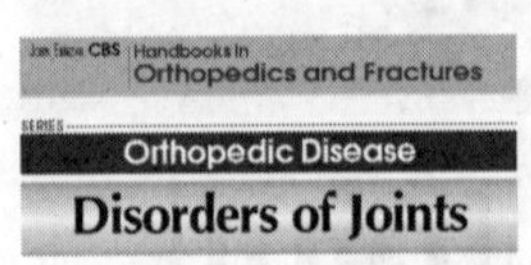

ISBN: 978-81-239-2110-5

First Edition: 2012

Published by Satish Kumar Jain and produced by Vinod K. Jain for
CBS Publishers & Distributors Pvt Ltd
4819/XI Prahlad Street, 24 Ansari Road, Daryaganj
New Delhi 110 002, India.
Website: www.cbspd.com
Ph: 23289259, 23266861, 23266867
e-mail: delhi@cbspd.com
Fax: 011-23243014
cbspubs@airtelmail.in.

Branches

- Bengaluru: Seema House 2975, 17th Cross, K.R. Road, Banasankari 2nd Stage, Bengaluru 560 070, Karnataka
  Ph: +91-80-26771678/79 Fax: +91-80-26771680 e-mail: bangalore@cbspd.com
- Pune: Bhuruk Prestige, Sr. No. 52/12/2+1+3/2 Narhe, Haveli (Near Katraj-Dehu Road Bypass), Pune 411 051, Maharashtra
  Ph: 020-64704058, 64704059, 32392277 Fax: +91-020-24300160 e-mail: pune@cbspd.com
- Kochi: 36/14 Kalluvilakam, Lissie Hospital Road, Kochi 682 018, Kerala
  Ph: +91-484-4059061-65 Fax: +91-484-4059065 e-mail: cochin@cbspd.com
- Chennai: 20, West Park Road, Shenoy Nagar, Chennai 600 030, Tamil Nadu
  Ph: +91-44-26260666, 26208620 Fax: +91-44-45530020 email: chennai@cbspd.com

Printed at Magic International, Greater Noida (UP)

to

---

my mother
(late) Sampath Kumari
who taught me that life is more than self and
there is more joy in giving and sharing than taking

my wife
Dr Parimala

my lovely children
Rakesh and Priyanka
who are an epitome of love, sacrifice, encouragement
and inspiration

all my teachers
who made me what I am today

all my students
past and present

and

all my patients

Dr John Ebnezar
is a legendary name as a prolific orthopedic writer. No other orthopedic surgeon in the world has come anywhere close to him in the number of books he has written in his field. He is the first orthopedic surgeon in the world to be listed in the **Guinness Book of World Records** for the most number of books written by an individual in a single year. For the same feat his name has been listed in the **India Book of Records.** This book, like all his previous books, carries his flavor of simple and lucid writing, excellent language, beautiful illustrations and excellent presentation of the topics. This book is a part of the 100+ book series he has brought out in a single calendar year of 2012 on a wide array of orthopedic problems of public health importance. No other individual in the world has brought out these many books in one year and this is a world record attempt. With these books he aims to educate the reader and the public about these common orthopedic problems.

All his books have been accepted very well and he has a great fan following all over the world. He has been bestowed with as many as 32 international, national and state awards including Karnataka state's highest civilian award the **Rajyotsava Award 2010** and the **Kempegowda Award 2011,** apart from the **Best Citizen of India Award** given by the International Publishing House. He is the pioneer in holistic orthopedics and is credited for discovering a new method of treatment for the common orthopedic problems and has done PhD in arthritis from the world famous S-VYASA University, Bangalore. He is currently president of the Neuro-Spinal Surgeons Association of India (Karnataka), the former Vice-President of the Indian Orthopedic Association, and is the founder president of various orthopedic bodies.

Preface

This book is a part of the 100$^+$ book series

JOHN EBNEZAR CBS Handbooks in Orthopedics and Fractures

which deals with the orthopedic problems of public health importance. The purpose of these books is to educate and create awareness among the readers about various problems associated with orthopedics. Through this way the readers get to know all about various orthopedic problems directly from a specialist. This will help a reader immensely in getting the right knowledge as most of them depend on the internet and magazines which distort and misrepresent various pieces of information concerning health topics, leaving the readers confused and worse still improperly educated. This may harm more than helping them find solutions to their problems. The purpose of these books, therefore, is to educate the readers right in their quest for knowledge on the common health and associated problems.

The 100$^+$ book series has been brought out in a single calendar year.

Orthopedic problems encountered by the people all over the world can be classified into two broad categories, traumatic and non-traumatic conditions. These problems are on the rise thanks to the increased instances of RTA's, natural calamaties, and rise in orthopedic life style problems. Among them, non-traumatic disorders affect a large section of the world population from a child to an old individual. This book deals with all the orthopedic joint disorders, some of which are common and some not so common. They come with their own unique set of problems. This is the first ever book which exclusively deals with the orthopedic joint problems and I have made an attempt to bring all the important basic aspects about these conditions in one book, so that the reader gets to know about them.

Highlights of this book

- Simple and lucid language
- Good illustrations

- Good clinical photographs wherever necessary
- Relevant X-rays
- Short summaries
- Anecdotes

This book has ubiquitous utility and usage and can be useful to the orthopedic surgeons, postgraduate students in orthopedics, undergraduate medical students, doctors from all disciplines of medicine, physiotherapists, therapists practising alternative systems of medicine, rehabilitation specialists, and most importantly the common people. It is particularly useful to those unsung heroes who work in remote areas with minimum infrastructure. They can use this book as a ready-reckoner. Seldom will you find a book that covers such a wide spectrum of readers.

Knowing about the orthopedic joint problems creates awareness about these conditions and helps one to understand them better and take the necessary preventive steps in preventing them from happening at the first place and if unfortunately, if one is a victim of these conditions, it helps them to know and understand everything about the cause, presentation, investigations and the treatment your doctor recommends for them.

Constructive criticism and useful suggestions are invited to make the book more effective in its forthcoming editions.

John Ebnezar

Acknowledgments

This volume is a part of the 100^{+} book series brought out in a single calendar year. This was a huge and mammoth task attempted first time ever by an author and a publisher in the world. Such an herculean effort could not have been possible without the active involvement of those concerned in CBS Publishers & Distributors. I thank Mr Satish K Jain, Managing Director of CBS P&D, for agreeing to be a part of this world-record feat in bringing out this book in the Series. My special thanks to Mr YN Arjuna who showed special interest in this work and channelized his entire energy into this improbable feat. My special thanks to Mrs Ritu Chawla and her entire dedicated team who have toiled day and night to make this dream a reality. I thank members of the entire editorial–production team of CBS P&D who have worked hard behind the scenes to bring out this book.

My special thanks to Dr Yogitha for actively helping me in the compilation of all the books. I also thank all the staff members of my hospital who have helped me at various levels during the making of this book.

John Ebnezar

Contents

John Ebnezar CBS | Handbooks in
Orthopedics and Fractures

TITLES IN THE SERIES

I Orthopedic Trauma

General Fractures

1 General Principles of Fractures and Dislocations
2 Fracture Treatment Methods
3 Fractures and their Complications
4 Atypical Fractures

Injuries of Upper Limb

5 Injuries of Shoulder
6 Injuries of Arm
7 Injuries of Elbow
8 Injuries of Forearm
9 Injuries of Wrist and Hand
10 Injuries of Distal Forearm and Wrist
11 Injuries of Hand
12 Injuries of Upper Limb

Injuries of Lower Limb

13 Injuries of Hip
14 Injuries of Femur
15 Injuries of Knee
16 Injuries of Knee and Leg
17 Injuries of Ankle and Leg
18 Injuries of Foot and Ankle
19 Injuries of Lower Limb

Injuries of Axial Skeleton

20 Injuries of Pelvis and Hip
21 Injuries of Spine
22 Injuries of Pelvis and Spine

23 Sports Injuries Volume I
24 Sports Injuries Volume II
25 Soft Tissue Problems in Orthopedics
26 Geriatric Trauma
27 Pediatric Trauma

II Orthopedic Disease

28 Congenital Orthopedic Problems
29 Developmental Orthopedic Problems

III Specific Orthopedic Problems

IV Regional Orthopedic Problems

V Orthopedic Injuries and Surgeries

VI Practical Examination

VII Orthopedic Problems of Different Ages

VIII Common Orthopedic Problems

IX Yoga Therapy in Common Orthopedic Problems

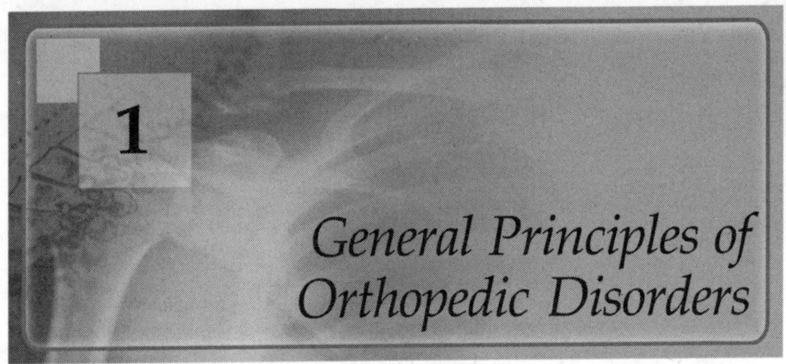

1 General Principles of Orthopedic Disorders

Introduction

Before discussing and knowing about various disorders of joints, let us try to know the general principles of various orthopedic disorders, how to diagnose them, all about deformities and their management and the broad principles of various treatment options from conservative to surgery in orthopedic disorders.

Arriving at a Diagnosis

Diagnosing orthopedic problems, involves taking proper history and conducting various clinical tests. We need to make a proper diagnosis. As in other branches of medicine, the diagnosis of orthopedic disorders revolves around the following fundamentals (Fig. 1.1). Therefore, we will try to discuss in brief the three steps of diagnosis in orthopedics.

History

History is "His- Story", as told by the patient. History taking is an art. Caution has to be exercised in the story "told" and the story "untold". Everything told should be taken with a pinch of salt lest the examiner is misled.

Certain Points of Importance in the History

Age: Certain diseases have predilection age groups, e.g. Perthes' disease and acute osteomyelitis are common in

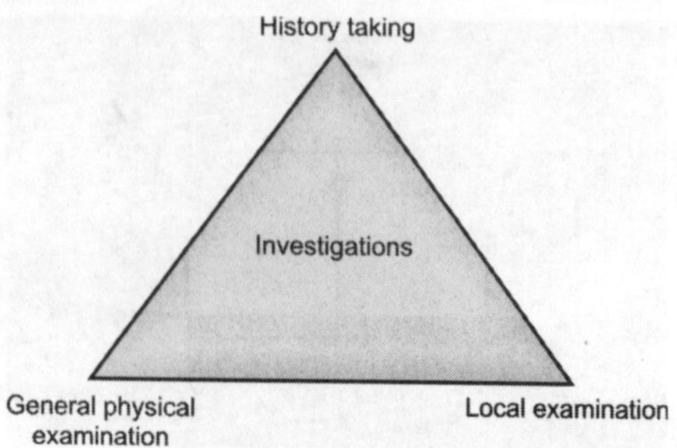

Fig. 1.1: Fundamentals of diagnosing orthopedic disorders

children. Avascular necrosis and degenerative disorders are common in the elderly. Some diseases may be seen in all the age groups, e.g. tuberculosis of bone and joints.

Quick facts: Age *vs.* orthopedic disease

< 1 year	Congenital dislocation of hip and cerebral palsy
1–2 years	Nutritional rickets
	Poliomyelitis
	Ewing's tumor
5–10 years	Tuberculosis of hip
	Perthes' disease
15–20 years	Slipped capital epiphysis
<15 years	Osteomyelitis
10–20 years	Bone malignancies
30–40 years	Rheumatoid arthritis
> 40 years	Degenerative disorders
	Prolapsed intervertebral disk (PIVD)
	Multiple myeloma, etc.

Sex: Congenital dislocation of hip (CDH) is common in females. Congenital talipes equinovarus (CTEV) is more common in males.

Quick facts—Sex *vs.* orthopedic disease

- *Males:* Perthes' slipped epiphysis, traumatic disorders, multiple myeloma, etc.
- *Females:* Rheumatoid arthritis, CDH, osteoporosis, etc.

Onset: It may be sudden or gradual.

Trauma: It could be a predisposing factor or the causative factor.

Traumatic points

Role of trauma vs. orthopedic disorders—trauma as a causative factor
- Fracture
- Dislocation
- Sprain
- Strain
- Subluxation

Trauma as a predisposing factor
- TB hip
- Perthes' disease
- Slipped capital epiphysis
- Osteogenic sarcoma
- Acute osteomyelitis, etc.

Fever: It may be high as in acute osteomyelitis or low grade as in tuberculosis.

Pain: This could be continuous or intermittent, low or high grade. One should be on guard about the radiating pains as these often mislead the examiner (Fig. 1.2).

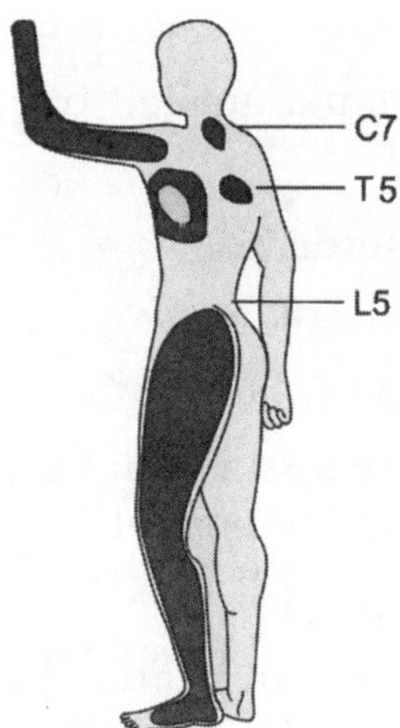

Fig. 1.2: Radiating pain at the upper limbs, chest and lower limbs

Facts—about radiating pains

Region	Radiation sites
Cervical spine	Shoulder, arm, forearm, and fingertips
Upper limbs	
a. Shoulder	Arm and elbow
b. Elbow	Forearm
Thoracic spine	Girdle pains
Lumbar spine	Groin, buttocks, posterior thigh, legs and foot
Hip knee.	

Any constitutional problems: Like weight loss, anorexia, etc. if present are a pointer towards neoplasm, tuberculosis, etc.

Seasonal variation: If present, it is suggestive of rheumatoid disorders. Apart from these points, relevant past history, socioeconomic status and personal history should be taken into account.

An attempt should be now made to place the problem into one of the following categories at the end of history taking.

Is the problem congenital?

If so, it will be present since birth or seen within a few years from birth. A strong family history is elicitable.

Is it developmental?

Here the disease is manifested during the process of development.

Is it an infective disorder?

History of fever, chills, rigors, sweating, etc. are present.

Is it inflammatory disorder?

Seasonal variation, remissions and exacerbation, multiple joint involvement, etc. are present.

Is it a metabolic disorder?

Nutrition, socioeconomic status, generalized skeletal disorder, etc. assume importance in this group.

Is it an endocrinal disorder?

Look for other evidences of hormonal imbalance, e.g.
Hypothyroidism → cretinism
Hypopituitarism → dwarf, etc.

Is it traumatic?

History of fall, road traffic accident (RTA), assault, etc. is elicited.

Is it degenerative?

Advancing age, slow progress is the hallmark.

Is it neoplastic?

Look for the features of either benign or malignant bone tumors.

If it cannot be categorized into any of the above, then it could be *idiopathic.* Having made a tentative diagnosis at the end of history, next important step is resorted to.

Diagnostic facts

• Present since birth	Congenital
• During the development process	Developmental
• History of fever, chills, rigors	Infective
• Nutrition, socioeconomic status	Metabolic
• Other evidences of Hormonal imbalance	Endocrinal
• Seasonal variation, multiple joint Involvement, etc.	Inflammatory
• H/o RTA, fall, assault	Traumatic
• Features of either benign Or malignant	Neoplastic
• Advancing age, etc.	Degenerative
• If no obvious complaints	Idiopathic

EXAMINATION

A good systematic clinical examination will help to clinch the diagnosis with certainty. *No sophisticated technology can replace the value of a good clinical examination.* A good clinician will make the diagnosis clinically and will make use of the investigation armamentarium judiciously. *A clinician should command the investigation and not vice versa.*

Examination of the locomotor system involves four steps.

STEP I

Examination of Gait

An examination of the gait is extremely important as it gives vital clues regarding the diagnosis.

Definition: It is a term used to describe the style of walking. This is dependent on not only normal muscles and joints but upon an intact central nervous system (CNS), peripheral nervous system and normal labyrinthine function.

Walking is divided into two phases.

The stance phase: This forms 60 percent of the gait and here the foot is on the ground (Figs 1.3A to C). It is further subdivided into:

- *Heel strike*—i.e. heel striking the ground.
- *Mid-stance*—here the foot is flat on the ground.
- *Push off*—here the foot is off the ground.

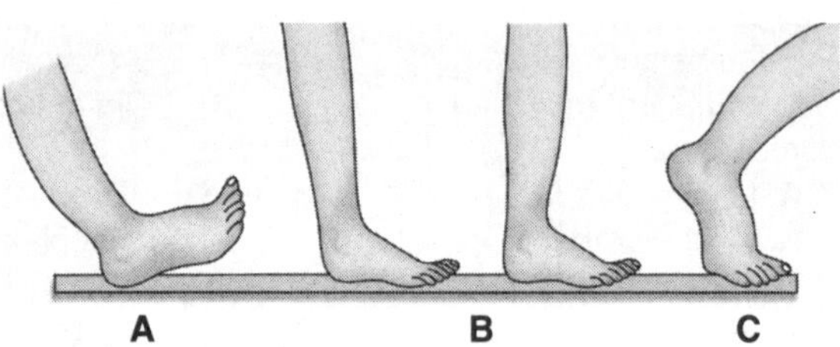

Figs 1.3A to C: Stance phase of gait: (A) Heel strike, (B) Midstance, (C) Push off

The swing phase: This forms 40 percent of the gait cycle and here the foot is not in contact with the ground (Figs 1.4A to C). It is further subdivided into:

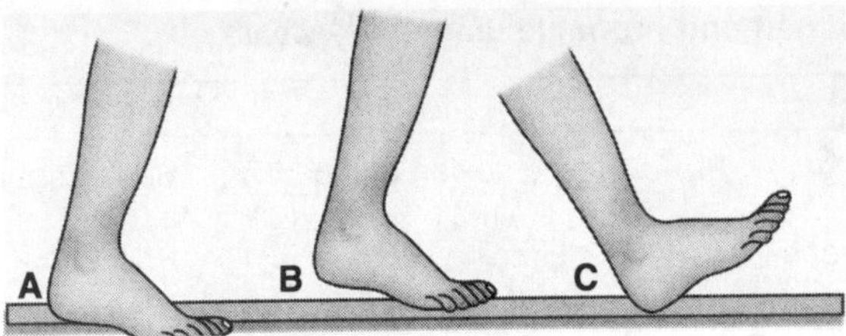

Figs 1.4A to C: Swing phase of gait: (A) Acceleration, (B) Swing through, (C) Deceleration

- *Acceleration*—here leg is in front of the body.
- *Swing through*—here leg continues to swing forward.
- *Deceleration*—swing slows down and the heel is ready for the strike.

In normal gait, each leg alternatively goes through a stance phase and a swing phase. Thus, the body is carried forward in normal walking by these rhythmic cycles.

Running gait: Here the sequences are the same as in walking but are faster.

Types of gait and probable diagnosis

Types	*What happens*	*Probable diagnosis*
Antalgic gait	Duration of stance phase decreased	Any painful lesion of foot, knee, hip, etc.
Gluteus medius gait	Lurch of body towards the affected side during every stance phase.	Paralysis of gluteus medius
Gluteus maximus gait	Backward lurch	Anterior polio
High stepping gait	To clear the dropped foot from the ground	Foot drop
Scissors gait	Legs cross while walking	Cerebral palsy
Short leg gait	When shortening > 2"	Limb shortening (congenital or acquired)

Contd.

Types of gait and probable diagnosis *(Contd.)*

Types	*What happens*	*Probable diagnosis*
Stiff hip gait	No flexion at hip	Septic arthritis at hip
Quadriceps gait	Limping gait with the hand On the knee	Polio
Trendelenburg gait	Pelvis drops on opposite side of the hip	Congenital or old traumatic dislocation of hip joint, nonunion fracture neck of femur
Calcaneus gait	No push off	Calf weakness
Stiff knee gait	Pelvis raised during swing phase	Stiff knee
Ataxic gait	Child walks with legs apart	Spinal cerebellar ataxia
Hysterical gait	Seen in conversion hysteria	

STEP II

General Physical Examination

A good general physical examination (GPE) from head to toe gives vital clues in the diagnosis of most of the orthopedic disorders, particularly generalized disorders of the skeleton, for example

- Metabolic disorders, e.g. rickets.
- Developmental disorders, e.g. osteogenesis imperfecta.

STEP III

Clinical Examination

Symptoms

The following are the usual presenting symptoms in a patient with orthopedic disorder.

Pain: This is the first and the most common complaint. It is a highly subjective complaint and can be classified as mild, moderate or severe.

The must-ask questions regarding the pain are how did it start? Is it related to trauma? Site of pain? Does it radiate? What are the aggravating and relieving factors? Does it interfere with sleep? etc.

Swelling: It may precede or follow pain. Relevant questions to be asked are site of the swelling, painful or painless. Is it rapidly growing (e.g. malignancy) or slow growing (benign growth)? Is it associated with fever, chills, etc. (e.g. infective origin), single or multiple (e.g. neurofibromas)?

Deformity: Sudden onset of deformity is usually seen in fresh fractures and dislocations. Longstanding deformities are usually seen in old fractures and other nontraumatic disorders like congenital, developmental, and metabolic conditions. The patient may complain of cosmetic and functional impairment due to the deformity.

Limitations of joint movements: In the initial stages, it may be due to muscle spasm; and in the later stages, it may be due to intra-articular adhesions (e.g. TB, septic arthritis, rheumatoid arthritis) or extra-articular contractures (like postburn contractures, Volkmann's ischemic contracture, etc.).

Limp: This could be painful (e.g. arthritis of hip, trauma) or painless (e.g. CDH, coxa vara). The patient may complain of difficulty or alteration in various day-to-day activities like walking, squatting, running, working, etc.

Limb weakness: This may be due to disuse atrophy, motor problems like polio, motor neuron disease, etc. muscle problems like muscular dystrophies, etc. or due to peripheral or diabetic neuropathies.

Signs

General: Look for the signs of anemia, fever, weight loss, etc.

Local

Deformity: Deformity may be due to an abnormality of bone or joint. If a joint is out of its anatomical position, a deformity is said to exist. In addition, in case of bone, deviation from its normal anatomy is deformity. In cases of old fractures and dislocations, the deformity may be fixed.

Remember

A fixed deformity is the angle between the neutral position of the normal joint and the position the deformed joint will reach.

Temperature: This is always compared with the normal side. Check with dorsum of the hand, as this is the most sensitive part.

Tenderness: This is elicited by examining from the normal to the affected area and is graded I to IV (Fig. 1.5).

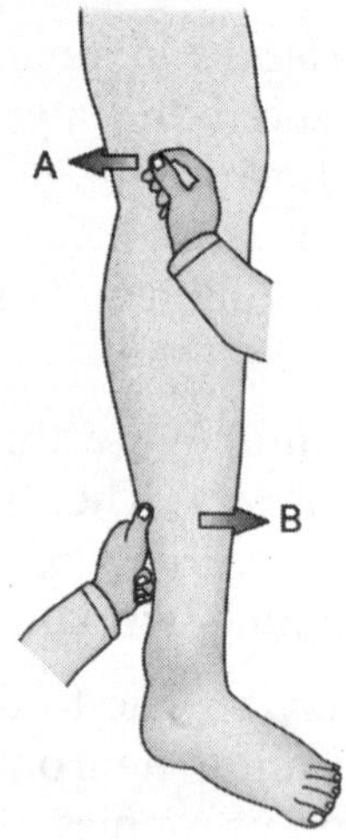

Fig. 1.5: Method of eliciting joint: (A) Line tenderness, (B) bony tenderness

Swelling: The following things are noted in the examination of a swelling.

- Decide the anatomical plane. The plane of the swelling could be either bone (swelling decreases in size when muscle is put into contraction) or could be in the muscle (swelling slightly decreases in size and gets fixed on muscle contraction) or could be between the muscle and the skin (no change in the size at the swelling when muscle is put into contraction). Also, examine the level of the swelling and identify whether it is epiphyseal, metaphyseal or diaphyseal (Figs 1.6A to D).
- Describe the shape as globular, oval or round, etc.
- Grade the consistency (*see* below).
- Decide whether it is congenital, neoplastic, etc.

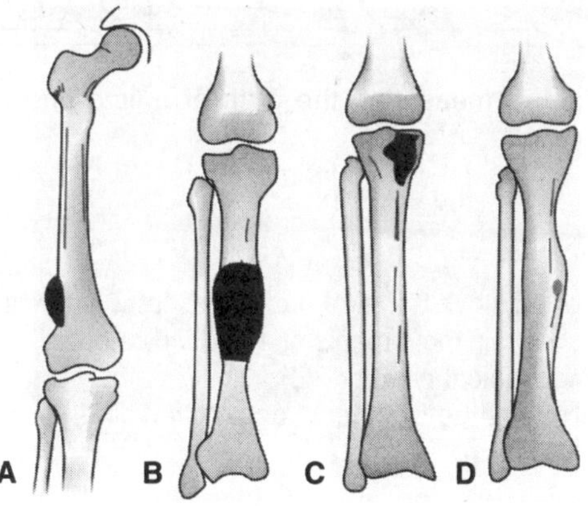

Figs 1.6A to D: Different levels of bony swelling: (A) Metaphyseal, (B and D) Diaphyseal, (C) Epiphyseal

- Look for slipping sign, sign of emptying, indentation sign and expansile impulse.

Remember

Grading of consistency

- Grade I — Very soft (like jelly).
- Grade II — Soft (as relaxed muscle).
- Grade III — Firm (like a contracted muscle).
- Grade IV — Hard (as a contracted biceps).
- Grade V — Stony and bone hard.

Movements of joint

- Active movement the patient himself moves the joint in one direction and later in the other. The extent of active movement is noted. Both the joints should be tested.
- Passive movement of the joint is tested by the examiner without causing pain. The extent of passive movement is noted (Fig. 1.7).

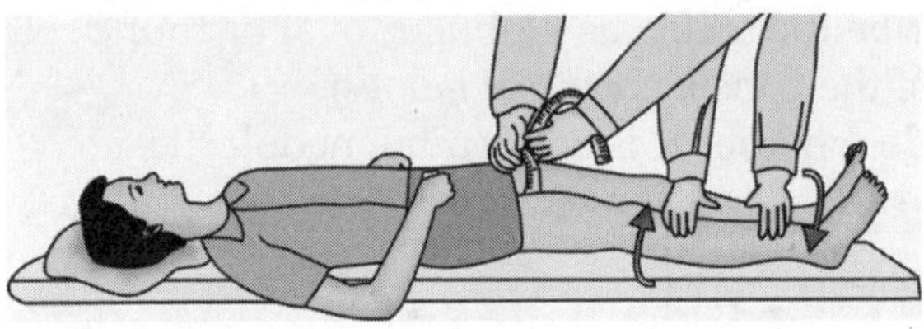

Fig. 1.7: Method of measuring the girth of a limb and checking the movements

Remember

- Limitation of all movements of a joint indicates arthritis.
- Limitation of certain movements of a joint indicates an extra-articular lesion or mechanical block.
- If passive movements exceed active movements, paralysis of muscle is likely.

Measurements: Accurate limb length measurements give vital clues regarding the diagnosis. Measurement should be taken for two purposes.

To know the limb length: For this, measurement is taken between two fixed bony points and is always compared with the normal.

Upper limbs

- *Arm length:* From the angle of acromion to the lateral epicondyle of humerus (Fig. 1.8).
- *Forearm length:* From the lateral epicondyle of humerus to the radial styloid process.

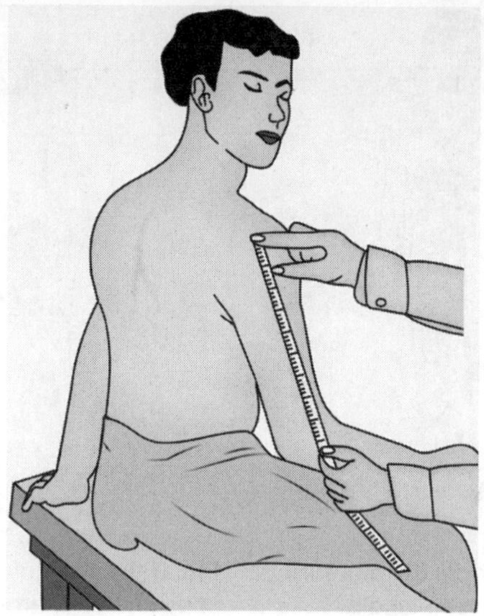

Fig. 1.8: Method of upper arm length measurement

Lower limbs

- *Thigh length:* From anterosuperior iliac spine to the medial knee joint line.
- *Leg length:* From the medial knee joint line to the medial malleolus.

To know the apparent length of the lower limbs measurement is taken from the xiphisternum to the medial malleolus (Fig. 1.9).

To know the girth of the limb: To detect wasting of muscles, the circumference of the limb is measured at fixed points on both sides, e.g. 18 cm above joint line in the thigh (Fig. 1.7).

Irregular thickening of bone and persistent discharging sinus: If this is present along with scars fixed to bone, it indicates chronic osteomyelitis (see box for causes of persistent sinus) (Fig. 1.10).

Peripheral, vascular and nervous system examination should be done next. This is discussed in appropriate sections.

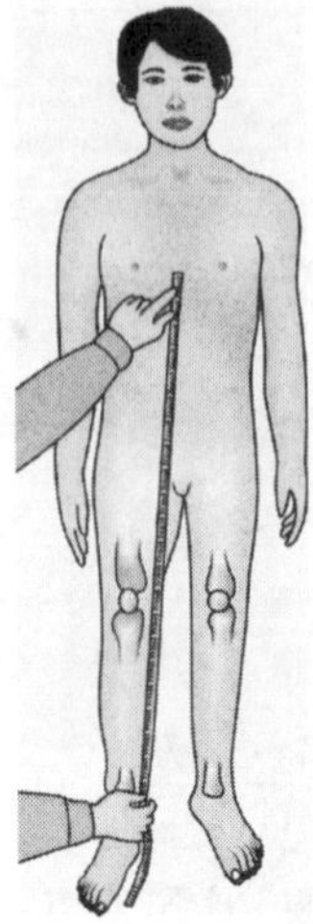

Fig. 1.9: Method of measuring apparent lower limb length

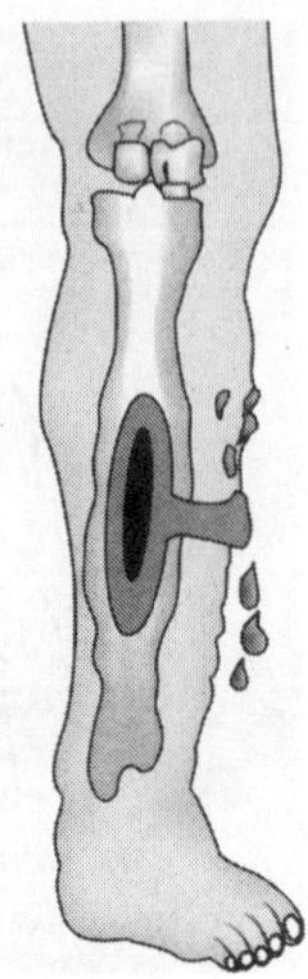

Fig. 1.10: Irregular thickening of bone and discharging sinus due to chronic osteomyelitis

Quick facts—sinus tracts

Causes of persistent discharging sinus:

- Unobliterated cavities.
- Unabsorbed sequestra.
- Epithelialization of sinus tract.
- Presence of foreign body.
- Secondary infection.
- Diabetes, steroid therapy, etc.
- Malignant change in the sinus.

INVESTIGATIONS

These help to confirm the diagnosis and in some cases help to make the diagnosis (e.g. crack fracture can be diagnosed only by X-ray). One has to choose carefully from the following vast armamentarium:

Laboratory investigation: This consists of blood investigations like routine hemogram, urine examination, ECG, chest X-ray, etc.

Special investigations:

- *Radiography:* At least two views of the affected part should be taken: oblique views and some special views are required in some cases.
- *CT scan:* Study the cross-section of the limb anatomy and bones.
- *MRI:* This is the recent gold standard in the investigative armamentarium of bone disorders. It helps to study the bone, soft tissues, medullary spread, etc. with greater accuracy. The only problem is its prohibitive cost.
- *Angiography and biopsy* help in tumor diagnosis.

Thus, a reasonably accurate diagnosis can be made by following the guidelines discussed above.

Steps in the process of diagnosis	
At the end of investigation	Final
At the end of examination	Provisional
At the end of history	Guess

DEFORMITIES AND THEIR MANAGEMENT: GENERAL PRINCIPLES

Definition

Any deviation from the normal anatomy of a bone and joint is called a deformity.

Classification

The deformities can be classified as shown in the box:

Acquired deformities are more commonly encountered than the congenital variety.

DEFORMITIES SINCE BIRTH (CONGENITAL)

These are due to some genetic abnormalities or environmental variations or both. They may be obvious at birth or may be seen a few years later. Incidence is around 2–3 percent. They may be so severe that the child is stillborn or may be so minor that it is not noticeable.

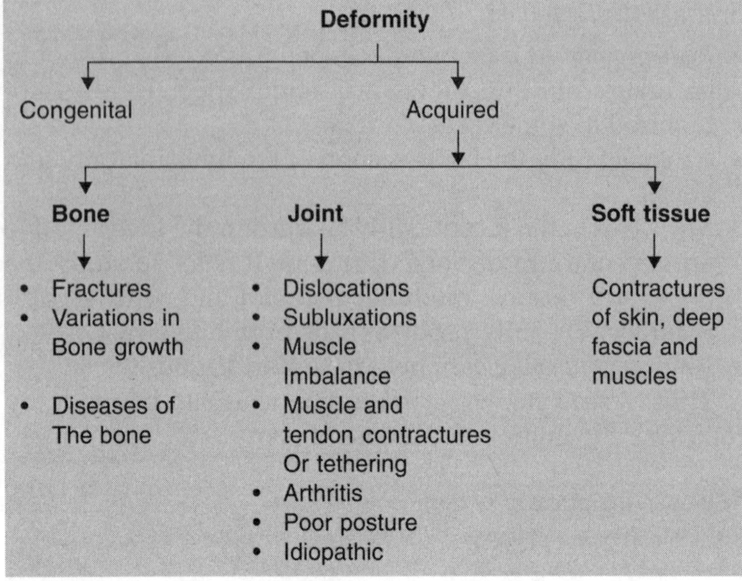

ACQUIRED DEFORMITIES

These could be due to problems in the bone, joint or soft tissues (Figs 1.11A to G).

Clinical facts: Famous orthopedic deformities due to fractures

• S-shaped deformity	Supracondylar fracture humerus
• Gunstock deformity	Malunited supracondylar fracture humerus
• Cubitus valgus fracture of humerus	Malunited lateral condyle
• Dinnerfork deformity	Malunited Colles
• Mallet finger	Avulsion tip of base of distal phalanx
• Genu varum/valgus	Tibial condylar fractures
• Varus-valgus at ankle	Ankle injuries
• External rotation Lower limb	Fracture neck femur, trochanteric fracture, fracture Shaft femur, fracture tibia.

BONE CAUSES

The following causes are responsible for deformities in the bone.

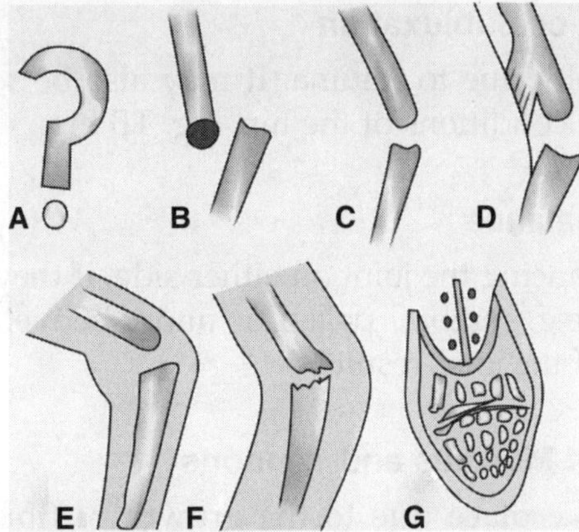

Figs 1.11A to G: Causes for deformity: (A) Idiopathic, (B) Dislocation, (C) Muscle imbalance, (D) Muscle tethering, (E) Soft tissue contractures, (F) Fractures, and (G) Postural

Growth Disturbances

Tumor, infections or trauma near the growth epiphysis can cause unequal stimulus, suppression or stimulation of growth. This results in bending, shortening or lengthening of a bone respectively, e.g. osteomyelitis, epiphyseal injuries, tumor.

Bone Disorders

Endocrine disorders, metabolic disorders, developmental disorders are some of the examples with bone deformities.

Fractures

This is by far the most important cause for a bone deformity. All displaced and fresh fractures cause temporary deformity while malunion or nonunion of fractures lead to deformities later.

JOINT CAUSES

The causes for the deformities due to joint are varied.

Dislocation or Subluxation

This is usually due to trauma. It may also be seen due to pathological conditions of the hip, e.g. TB hip.

Muscle Imbalance

Muscles balancing the joint on either side, if they are either overactive (e.g. cerebral palsy) or under active, e.g. polio, deformity of the joint results.

Tethering of Muscles and Tendons

This can take place due to the growth of fibrous tissue following infections or due to callus following fractures. Tethering restricts the joint movements and if held for some time deformity results, e.g. VIC, tenosynovitis of finger flexors.

Arthritis

Any joint may give rise to muscle spasm in the initial stages and fibrous or bony ankylosis in later stages giving rise to deformities, e.g. TB knee, rheumatoid hand, TB hip.

Postural

This is due to improper postural habits like hallux valgus in women due to tight and rigid shoes.

Idiopathic

Here, there is no apparent cause for the joint deformities, e.g. idiopathic scoliosis.

SOFT TISSUE CAUSES

Soft tissue contractures (skin and deep fascia) other than the muscle contractures can also cause joint deformities, e.g. Dupuytren's contractures, post burn contracture.

Treatment Options

Conservative Measures

These include manipulative correction under anesthesia and retention by splints or casts, gradual correction by traction or splints, etc. (e.g. turn buckle splints). Correction by plaster wedging is hazardous.

Surgical Measures

There are various surgical options available:

- *Ilizarov:* This is the gold standard for deformity correction in recent times.
- Soft tissue release by surgical methods.
- Tenolysis, tendon lengthening or tendon transfers are successfully employed in polio, cerebral palsy, etc.
- *Arthroplasty* can be crude as a salvage procedure (e.g. girdle stone excision in TB hip) or sophisticated as in total hip replacement or total knee replacement in osteoarthritis, rheumatoid and other disorders.
- *Corrective osteotomy* this is a simple but effective procedure to correct joint deformities, e.g. French osteotomy in cubitus varus deformity.
- *Arthrodesis* fusion of the joints in functional positions in badly damaged joints, e.g. TB knee, rheumatoid arthritis.
- *Epiphyseal growth arrests:* When potential for growth is still left, stapling of the epiphysis can be attempted on one side to correct the bending deformity, e.g. in genu varum or valgum.

Now after having understood the basics of clinical examination and deformity management, let us know the broad principles and various options of treating orthopedic disorder.

TREATMENT OF ORTHOPEDIC DISORDERS: GENERAL PRINCIPLES

There are three time-tested and time-honored treatment methods: (i) masterly inactivity, (ii) conservative methods, and (iii) operative treatment methods of treating an orthopedic disorder.

Masterly Inactivity

It is interesting to observe that nearly 50 percent of the orthopedic disorders can be managed best by *not doing anything*. To allay the doubts, fears, myths, and misconceptions, a patient has regarding his ailment and assuring him that nothing is seriously wrong with him is all that is required.

This is more of a 'mind' management than 'orthopedic' management and is more a 'human' care than 'health care'!

Conservative Methods

This is the next commonly advocated and recommended method of treatment.

Rest

This implies not total rest but selective rest with avoidance of unnecessary activities and strain. HO Thomas first advocated this and of late due to improved methods of treatment and technology; emphasis is now on early restoration of activities and not passive rest.

Support

This enables the diseased part to heal, provides rest, prevents deformities, relieves pain and also supports the patients psychologically, e.g. plaster splints for fractured limbs, lumbosacral belts and corsets for low backache, calipers in polio, cervical collars for neck pains, knee cap, ankle binders, etc. (Figs 1.12 and 1.13).

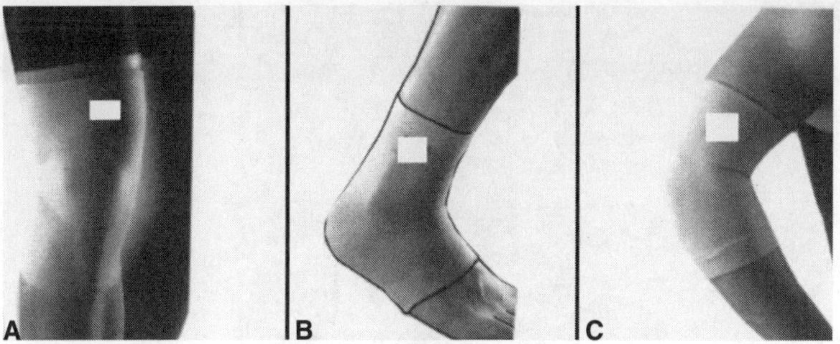

Figs 1.12A to C: Supportive braces: (A) Knee support cap, (B) Ankle support, (C) Elbow support

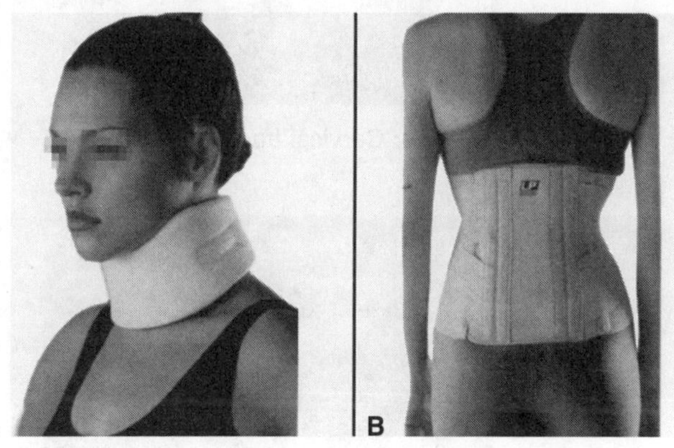

Figs 1.13A and B: Neck and back supports: (A) Cervical collar, (B) Sacrolumbar support

Traction

This is a popular method of treating certain chronic orthopedic conditions like low backache, cervical spondylosis, etc. In these conditions, it is known to reduce pain, muscle stiffness, spasm, etc. (Figs 1.14 and 1.15).

Physiotherapy

Physiotherapy, if properly understood and skillfully executed by trained persons, gives excellent results in

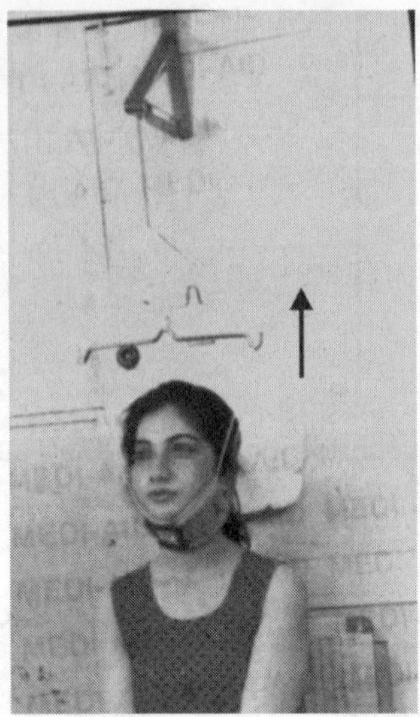

Fig. 1.14: Cervical traction

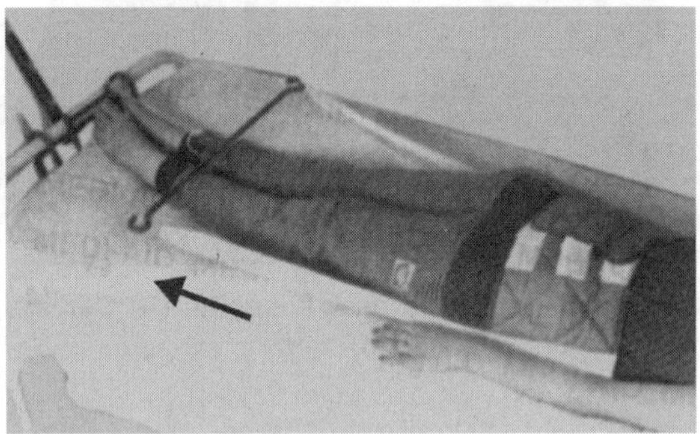

Fig. 1.15: Lumbar traction

treating orthopedic disorders and in postoperative rehabilitation. For optimum results, physiotherapy should be pursued systematically until its final logical conclusion and should not be abandoned in between. Physiotherapy has a great role to play and sometimes is the only treatment option in diseases like polio, cerebral palsy, hemiplegia, paraplegia, etc.

The following are the various physiotherapy options:

- *Active exercises:* Here the patient is made to actively contract his or her muscles and joints against resistance and weight. This helps to mobilize the joints, strengthen the muscles and to improve coordination or balance (Fig. 1.16).

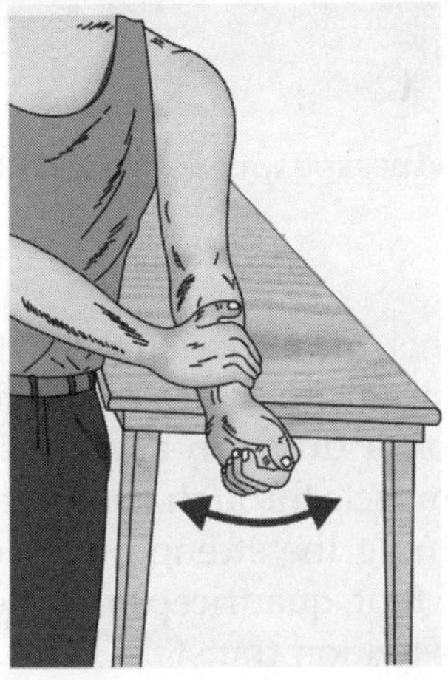

Fig. 1.16: Method of active wrist dorsal and palmar flexion of the wrist joint

- *Passive exercises:* This can be given by the physiotherapist normally or by machines which can provide continuous passive movements of the joints. This is of immense help to maintain the mobility of all the joints when active movements are not possible due to paralysis or injury to the muscles. Thus, the joints are kept supple and deformities are prevented (Fig. 1.17).

> *Note:* Active muscle strengthening exercise could be either isometric (here muscle does not move and hence no change in length, e.g. pushing against a static object) or isotonic (here muscle actually moves, e.g. quadriceps exercises).

- *Electrical muscle stimulation:* Depending upon whether the nerve supply of a muscle is intact or not, two types of electrical stimulation is chosen:

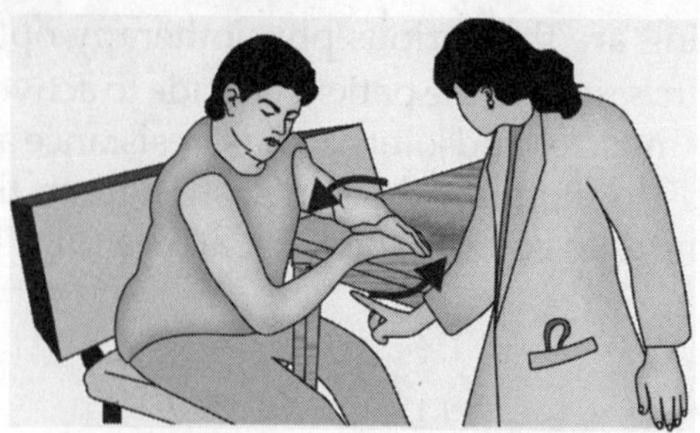

Fig. 1.17: Self-assisted passive wrist flexion and extension with the hand at the edge of a table

- *Faradism:* In this, the nerve supply of the muscle should be intact. In faradism, an electronic stimulator delivers shocks at shorter duration at a frequency of 1 mm at 50 Hg to the muscle through its intact motor nerve root, e.g. for regaining the strength of intrinsic muscles of the hand and foot, quadriceps muscle and to retain the tendons after tendon transfers.
- *Galvanism:* Here the muscle is stimulated directly with shocks of longer durations (100–1000 mm at frequency of 5–15 Hg). When the muscle is denervated after a peripheral nerve injury, etc. this treatment modality helps.

• *Hydrotherapy:* This is particularly useful in patients suffering from rheumatoid arthritis. The warmth and buoyancy of water helps to relieve pain and muscle spasm.

• *Heat therapy* by direct application of heat the local temperature underneath the tissues rises up to 10° inducing vasodilatation, reduced muscle spasm and decreased pain. There are two varieties of heat therapies.
  - *Surface heat:* This heats only the superficial tissues and consists of hot packs, infrared heat, paraffin wax bath, etc.
  - *Deep heat:* Apart from vasodilatation, it stimulates the circulatory mechanism and helps in heating the deeper structures. It is also helpful in treating joint disorders,

e.g. short-wave diathermy, ultrasound, interferential heat therapy (Fig. 1.18).

- *Manipulation:* This term denotes a deliberate attempt by the surgeon to passively move the joints bone or soft tissues. It is useful in three specific purposes:

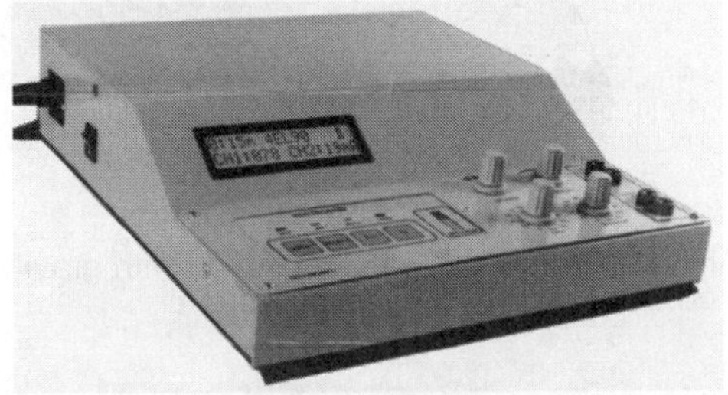

Fig. 1.18: Equipment for interferential therapy (IFT)

  - *Manipulation for correction of deformity:* Closed reduction of fractures and dislocations and manipulation of a clubfoot falls under this category. This is done under general anesthesia and after the correction; the part is immobilized in splints, etc. to retain the correction.
  - *Manipulation for joint stiffness:* This is useful in the knee joints; it may be successful in shoulder and foot but responds poorly in cases of elbow and hand. The manipulation should be done gradually under general anesthesia and forcible or abrupt movements should be avoided (Fig. 1.19).
  - *For relief of chronic pain:* Manipulation may help in chronic pain of shoulder tarsal, spine or sacroiliac joints.

Note: Manipulation should not be done in acute painful conditions for fear of aggravating the problem.

Massage: Delicate, continuous and systematic massage if done regularly has a lot of beneficial effects like relief of pain, smoothening effect, etc. (Fig. 1.20).

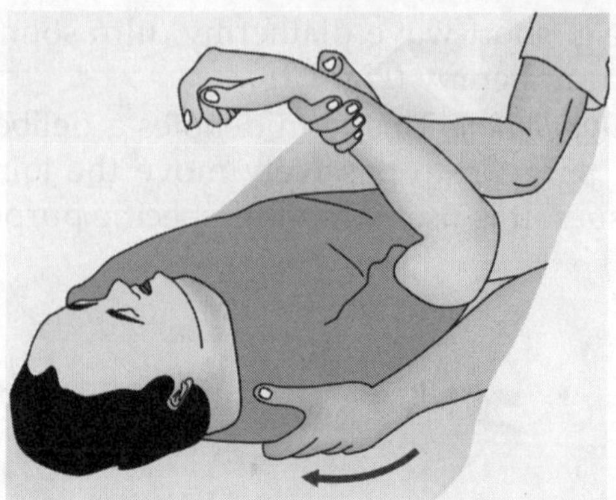

Fig. 1.19: Active assisted shoulder abduction with gravity eliminated

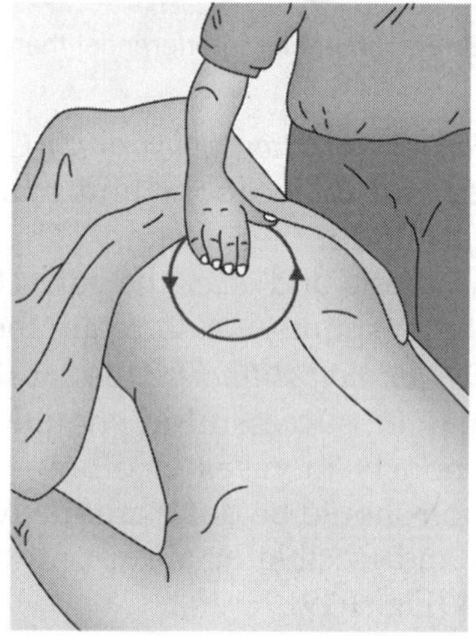

Fig. 1.20: Technique of back massage

Radiotherapy

It has a role in:

- *Inflammatory conditions* like recalcitrant ankylosing spondylitis.
- *Neoplastic conditions,* e.g. Ewing's sarcoma and giant cell tumor recurrence.

Drugs

Drugs though limited have an important role to play in orthopedic practice. The commonly used ones are:

- *Analgesics and anti-inflammatory agents:* These help relieve pain and inflammation. Long-acting drugs are preferred in chronic disorders like rheumatoid arthritis, etc. while short-acting drugs are preferred in acute infections, trauma, etc.
- *Muscle relaxants:* These are useful to relieve painful muscle spasms.
- *Sedatives and anxiolytics:* These are used to induce sleep, alleviate anxiety and to relieve muscle spasm.
- *Antibiotics* these are extremely useful in acute and chronic infections of bones and joints. Broad-spectrum, bactericidal agents are usually preferred.
- *Hormones:* Growth hormones, stilbestrol for metastatic carcinomas, anabolic steroids and estrogens for osteoporosis are some of the examples.
- *Specific drugs:* Vitamin C for scurvy, vitamin D for rickets is some of the examples.
- *Cytotoxic drugs:* These are used as chemotherapeutic agents for malignant tumors.

OPERATIVE TREATMENT METHODS

Operative treatment should be resorted after great deliberations and when all other treatment options have been tried or thought of. Once undertaken, it should not worsen the condition of the patient.

A brief account of various orthopedic surgical techniques is presented here.

Osteotomy (Figs 1.21A and B)

This is a procedure of creating a surgical fracture to achieve the following objectives:

- To correct excessive angulations, bowing or rotation of a long bone.

- To compensate and correct the malalignment of a joint.
- To correct leg length inequality either by shortening or by lengthening.
- To alter the line of weight bearing and increase the stability at the hip joint, e.g. abduction osteotomy.
- To relieve the pain in an arthritic hip, e.g. displacement osteotomy, high tibial osteotomy (Fig. 1.22).

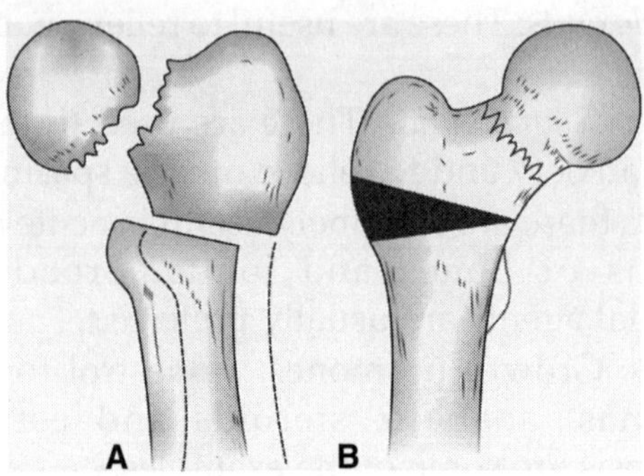

Figs 1.21A and B: Different types of osteotomies: (A) McMurray's displacement osteotomy, (B) Angulation osteotomy

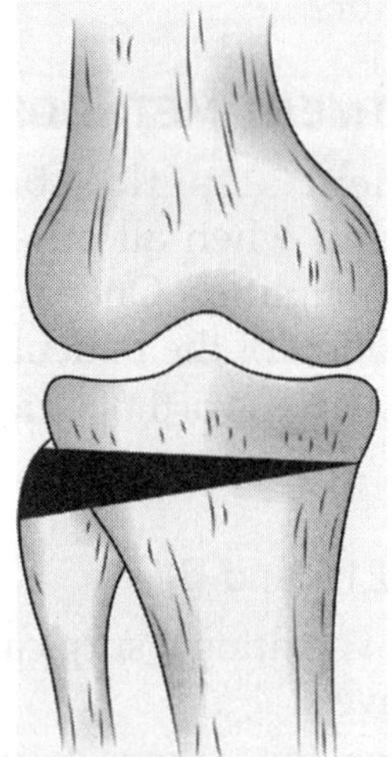

Fig. 1.22: High tibial osteotomy done in OA knee

A quick glance at famous osteotomies

Upper limbs	*Done for*
• French osteotomy	Malunited supracondylar Fracture humerus
• Fernandez and Campbell Osteotomy	Malunited Colles' fracture
Lower limbs	
• Salter, Chiari, Pemberton	CDH
• McMurray's, Shanz	Fracture neck femur
• Pauwel's	OA Hip
• High tibial osteotomy	OA Knee
• Dwyer's osteotomy	Clubfoot
Spinal osteotomy	Ankylosing spondylitis

Arthrodesis

Arthrodesis is fusion of the joints by surgical methods. Because it limits the function of the joint, arthroplasty it is more commonly used nowadays. However, it can be used in the following situations:

- Gross destruction of the joints as in rheumatoid arthritis, Charcot's joints or advanced osteoarthritis.
- Quiescent tubercular arthritis.
- Gross instability due to muscle paralysis as in polio.
- For permanent correction of a deformity.

Methods

There are three methods:

Intra-articular Arthrodesis

Here joint is opened, articular cartilage is denuded, cancellous bone grafts are packed, joint is kept in a functional position and fixed either internally or externally by plaster, etc. (Fig. 1.23).

Extra-articular Arthrodesis

This is indicated in infective condition of the hip, shoulder or spine. In this, there is no risk of reactivating or spreading the infection as the joint itself is not opened, but bone-to-bone fusion is obtained above or below the joint.

Combined Arthrodesis

This is a combination of the above two procedures.

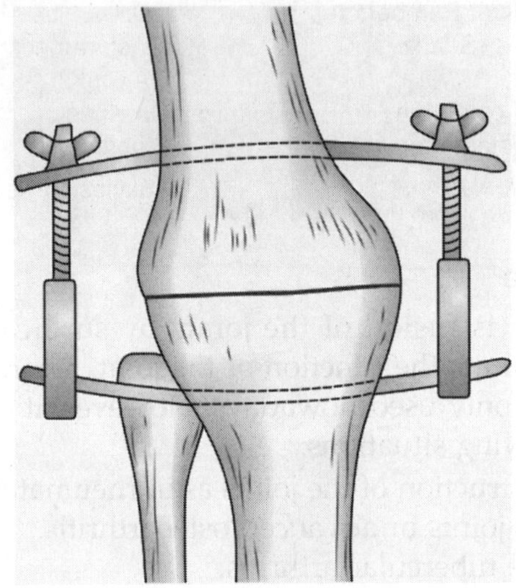

Fig. 1.23: Charnley's compression arthrodesis

> *Note:* Arthrodesis of a joint gives it stability but takes away its mobility. It is like robbing Peter to pay Paul.

Arthroplasty

Arthroplasty is an operation to construct a new mobile joint. The following are the indications:

- Advanced osteoarthritis or rheumatoid arthritis of hip, knee, shoulder, elbow, hand and foot.
- Quiescent destructive tuberculous arthritis of hip and elbow.
- Fracture neck nonunion in patients of more than 60 years.
- Rarely to correct deformity, e.g. hallux valgus.

Practical facts: Arthrodesis

Each joint should be fixed in its functional position as mentioned below to enable the patient to continue using it:

Joints	*Functional positions*
Upper limbs	
Shoulder	30° Abd/30° flexion/40° internal rotation
Elbow	
• Eating hand (right)	90° of flexion
• Toilet hand (left)	70° of flexion
Wrist	20° dorsiflexion
Forearm	10° pronation
MP joint	35° flexion
IP joints	45° flexion
Lower limbs	
Hip	15° flexion, no adduction or abduction or rotation
Knee	20° flexion
Ankle (men)	90° or neutral position
• Ankle (women)	15–20° of plantar flexion
Metatarsophalangeal Joints of big toe	Slight extension

Types

There are three varieties of arthroplasties (Figs 1.24 and 1.25) namely:

- *Excision arthroplasty:* Here one or both the articular surfaces are excised; fibrous tissue fills up in the gap thus created and provides mobility (Fig. 1.24A). It is usually done in hip, elbow and metatarsophalangeal joint of the great toe.
- *Hemireplacement arthroplasty:* Either of the articulating surfaces is removed or replaced by prosthesis of similar shape and size, e.g. Austin Moore's prosthesis in fracture neck nonunion (Fig. 1.24B).
- *Total replacement arthroplasty:* Here both the articular surfaces are excised and replaced by prosthetic components, the larger joint is replaced by a metallic prosthesis, and the smaller joint by high-density

polyethylene (Fig. 1.24C). Both the components are fixed by acrylic cement, e.g. total hip replacement for osteoarthritis or rheumatoid hip and partial or total knee replacement for advanced intractable osteoarthritis or rheumatoid arthritis (Figs 1.25 to 1.27).

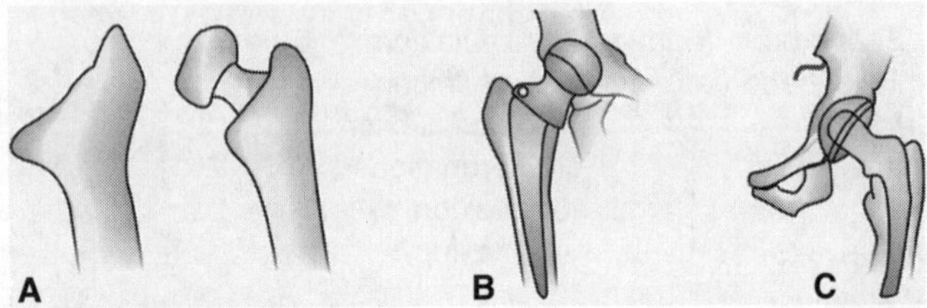

Figs 1.24A to C: Different types of arthroplasties: (A) Excision arthroplasty, (B) Hemireplacement arthroplasty, (C) Total hip replacement

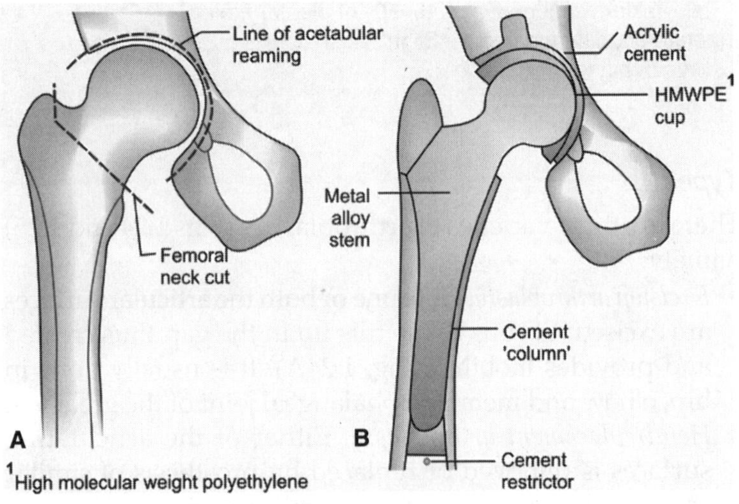

Figs 1.25A and B: Cemented total hip replacement

Bone Grafting Operations

Bone grafting is used in the following situations in orthopedic practice:

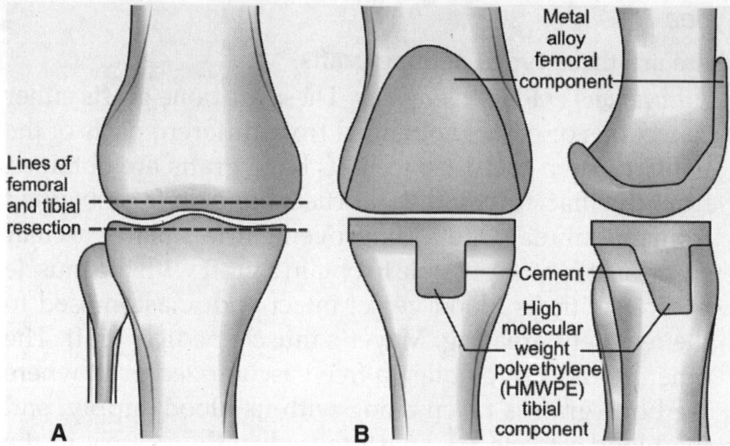

Figs 1.26A and B: Cemented total knee replacement

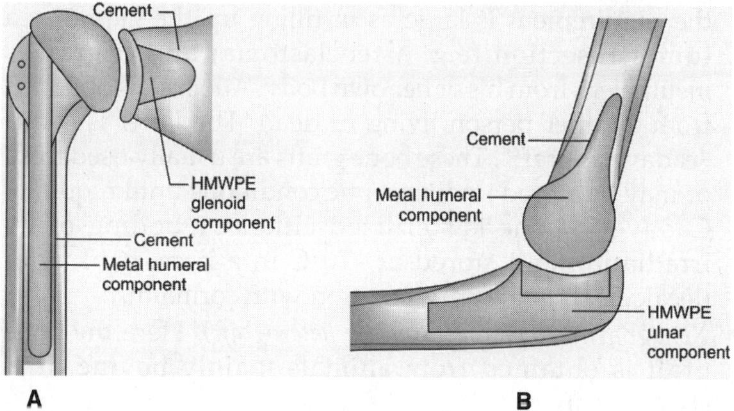

Figs 1.27A and B: (A) Unconstrained total shoulder replacement, (B) Unconstrained total elbow replacement

- To promote union in cases of nonunion or ununited fractures.
- In arthrodesis of joints for intraarticular or extra-articular fusion.
- To fill a defect or cavity in a bone.

Types

There are three types of bone grafts.

- *Autogenous grafts or autografts:* These are bone grafts either cancellous or cortical obtained from different parts of the patient's own body. Cancellous bone grafts are obtained from the iliac crest and the cortical bone graft is obtained from the fibula. Due to improvement in micro vascular surgery, it is now possible to obtain a graft with the muscle pedicle with its blood vessel intact and anastomosed to the recipient area, e.g. Meyer's muscle pedicle graft. The other method is to obtain a free vascularized graft where the bone graft is taken along with its blood supply, and the blood vessels are anastomosed to the vessels in the recipient area, e.g. fibula with its blood supply intact.
- *Allograft or homograft or homogeneous grafts:* Here the bone graft is obtained from another person's body usually if the requirement is large as in filling up the gap after a tumor resection (e.g. osteoclastoma) and if graft is insufficient from his or her own body. Allograft is obtained from another person living or dead. The latter is called "cadaveric graft". These bone grafts are usually used fresh or may be stored under aseptic conditions until required. Cadaveric bone is sterilized either by boiling or by irradiation and stored at –70°C in a bone bank after decalcification and preservation with formalin.
- *Xenografting (heterogeneous or heterograft):* Here the bone graft is obtained from animals mainly bovine. It is sparingly used.

Artificial bone: This is made up of hydroxyapatite and is now being used in some centers.

Role of a Bone Graft

It provides a scaffold or a temporary bridge upon which a new bone is laid down. Thus, the bone cells of the graft die and are eventually replaced by a new living bone. Vascularized grafts are incorporated very rapidly.

Tendon Surgeries

This includes:

Tendon transfers: In this operation the insertion of a healthy functioning muscle is moved to a new site, so that it has a different action. Other intact tendons will take care of the original function of the transferred tendon.

Indications

- Muscle paralysis as in polio or peripheral nerve injury.
- Muscle imbalance as in cerebral palsy.
- In rupture or cut tendon where direct suture is not possible.

Tendon grafting: In this, a length of free tendon is used to bridge a gap between the severed ends of the recipient tendon, e.g. reconstruction of flexor tendons severed in the fibrous digital sheaths of the hand.

Free tendon graft is usually obtained from the Palmaris longus or from one of the toe extensors at the dorsum of the foot (Fig. 1.28).

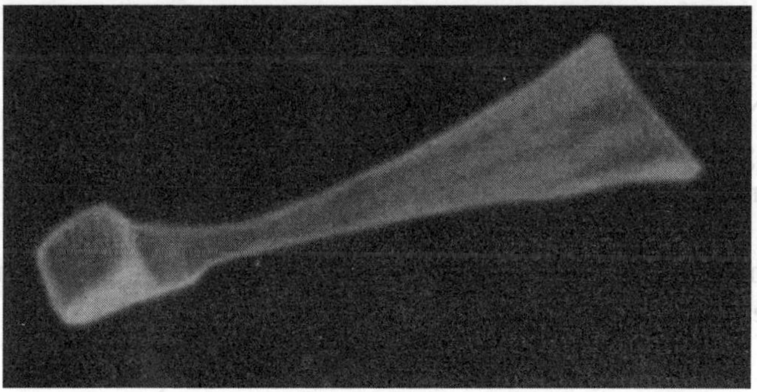

Fig. 1.28: Tendon graft

Equalization of leg length: In patients with unequal leg length as in polio, equalization of leg length can be obtained by:

- Leg lengthening by Ilizarov's technique.
- Leg shortening, especially in femur or tibia. Not advocated as a routine procedure.
- Arrest of epiphyseal growth by stapling in children.

A Quick Recap

Treatment method in orthopedics

Masterly inactivity

Conservative methods:
- Rest
- Support
- Traction
- Physiotherapy
- Radiotherapy
- Massage
- Drugs

Operative methods:
- Osteotomy
- Arthrodosis
- Arthroplasty
- Bone graft procedures
- Tendon surgeries
- Equalization of leg length
- Excision of tumors
- Amputations

Now after having understood the general principles of diagnosis in orthopedics, approach to a patient and general principles of management in orthopedic disorders, let us now try to understand the various disorders of joints that are common and let us get ourselves familiarized with its presentation and treatment methods.

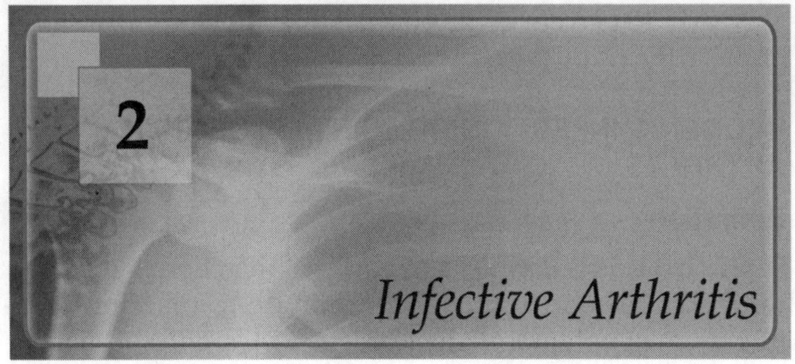

This chapter deals with important infective joint problems in orthopedics

Introduction

Arthritis is a non-specific term denoting acute or chronic inflammation of the joint. Clinically, arthritis falls into the following groups:

Osteoarthritis

- Primary
- Secondary

Rheumatoid arthritis

- Adult
- Juvenile

Infective arthritis

- Acute
- Chronic

Metabolic arthritis

- Gout
- Pseudogout

Nonspecific monoarthritis

Neuropathic joint disorders, e.g. Charcot's

Special forms:

- Hemophilic arthritis
- Psoriatic arthritis
- Psychogenic arthritis.

Nearly 10 percent of the population suffers from one form of the arthritis or the other.

PYOGENIC INFECTION OF JOINT OR SEPTIC ARTHRITIS

Definition

Septic arthritis is defined as a bacterial infection of the joint, which causes an intense inflammatory reaction with migration of polymorph nuclear leucocytes, and subsequent release of proteolytic enzymes. This could lead to destruction of the articular cartilage and later the joint.

Do you know?

Newer definition of septic arthritis.
A positive synovial fluid culture or a synovial fluid WBCs count of greater than 50,000 with 75 percent polymorphic neutrophils and a negative lyme titer.

Causative Organisms

The most common offending organisms are *Staphylococcus aureus* (50%), *Streptococcus* (20%), *Pneumococcus* (10%), *Gonococcus, E. coli,* etc. *H. influenzae* is very common in children less than 2 years. *Blood culture is positive only in 60 percent of cases.*

Routes of entry for organisms: 5 Ps

Primary focus is in RS, GIT, etc.
Pyogenic osteomyelitis
Punctured wounds
Pneumonia, typhoid, etc.
Primary focus within the joint, absent in few.

Predisposing Factors

The following act as predisposing factors: trauma, diabetes, steroid therapy, malignancy, etc.

Sites of Involvement of the Joint

In adults

- Knee (53%)
- Hip (20%)
- Elbow (17%)
- Shoulder (10%)

In children

- Knee (39%)
- Hip (32%)

Remember

Ninety percent of cases of septic arthritis are monarticular and 10 percent are polyarticular.

Pathology

The following pathological events take place:

Exudation into joint: This could be serous, serofibrinous or purulent depending upon the severity of infection.

Destruction of articular cartilage by plasmin, cathepsin, prostaglandins, etc.

Capsules, ligaments are destroyed by pus.

Clinical Features

Septic arthritis usually presents as monarticular affection in 90 percent and polyarticular in 10 percent of cases and fever is seen in only 50 percent of the cases. Limp is a common complaint. The severity of clinical manifestation depends upon the severity of disease (Table 2.1).

Investigations

Joint Aspirate and Synovial Fluid Analysis

This is the most accurate diagnostic tool for septic arthritis. The synovial fluid is tested for cells, sugar and proteins. Gram staining is positive in 60 percent of the cases for gram-positive cocci.

Table 2.1: Types of septic arthritis

Serous	*Serofibrinous*	*Purulent*
• Pain is less • Movements of the joint ↓ • Local temperature ↑ • Flexion deformity	• Tenderness +ve • Fever +ve • Night pains +ve	• Patient is very ill • Pain +ve • Wasting +ve • Temperature ↑

Note: Nearly one-third of patients affected with bacterial arthritis suffer loss of joint function.

Laboratory Investigations

WBCs (polymorphs) are raised to 50,000–1,00,000 (80% of cases), ESR increased more than 20 mm/hr (in 50% of cases), Hb percentage decreases. Blood culture is positive in 35–50 percent of the cases. CRP should be done within 24 hours of presentation.

The importance of C-reactive protein (Negative predictor)

If the CRP is < 10 mg/dl, the probability that the patient does not have septic arthritis is 87 percent.

Radiographs

Early Stages

The earliest findings in the radiographs are soft tissue swelling and periarticular osteoporosis.

Late Stages

In the later stages, cartilage destruction, and loss of joint space, necrosis of bone (Figs 2.1A and B), epiphyseal disturbances, fibrous ankylosis, and bony ankylosis may be seen Figs 2.2A to C.

Treatment

Arthrotomy or joint drainage the joint is aspirated first, if pus is present, open arthrotomy is indicated. The pus is cultured and is subjected to Gram staining. Appropriate antibiotics

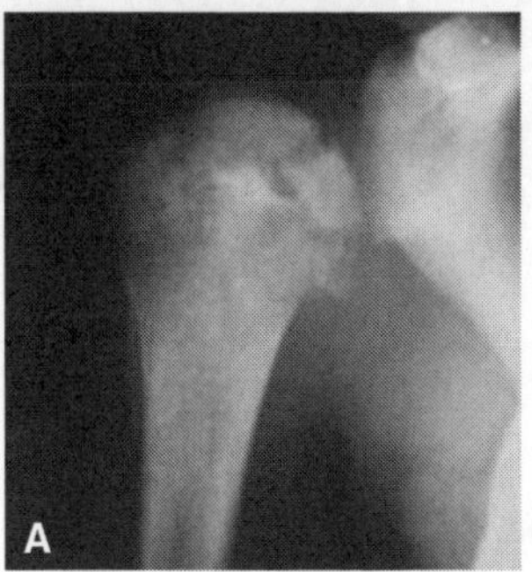

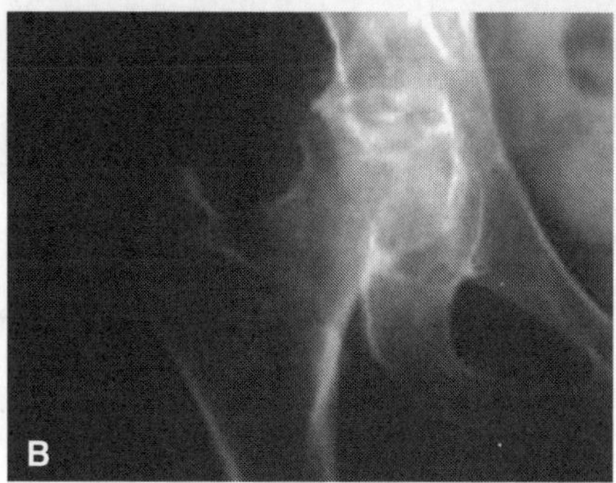

Figs 2.1A and B: (A) Septic arthritis of the shoulder, (B) Bony ankylosis hip due to septic arthritis

are then chosen and are given intravenously before surgical drainage. Antibiotics are used for a minimum period of 2–4 weeks.

Immobilization of the joints by using plaster of Paris splints in functional position reduces pain.

Radical treatment is reserved for all except, for very early cases, which do not respond rapidly within 24 hours to antibiotics and immobilization.

If cartilage is destroyed, aim for ankylosis in functional position by plaster casts.

Complications

- Joint destruction (Fig. 2.2B).
- Pathological dislocation.
- Osteoarthritis in later years.
- Ankylosis—fibrous or bony (Fig. 2.2C).
- Acute osteomyelitis.
- Amyloidosis very rarely develops.
- Septicemia, pyemia, etc.

Remember

Tom Smith arthritis is a septic arthritis of the hip joint seen in infants.

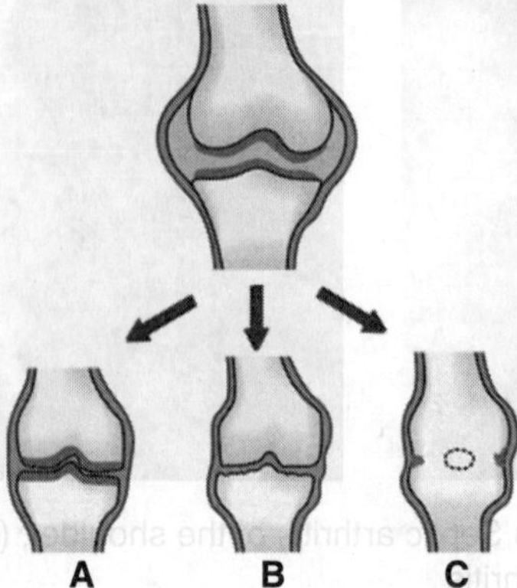

Figs 2.2A to C: Stages of septic arthritis: (A) Synovitis, (B) Arthritis, and (C) Bony ankylosis

Quick facts

- Sites of septic arthritis in parenteral drug abusers:
  - Sacroiliac joint
  - Sternal articulations
  - Pubic symphysis
- Organisms responsible are:
  - *Staphylococcus aureus*
  - *Pseudomonas aeruginosa*
  - *Serratia marcescens*
- In sickle cell anemia, *Salmonella* is the organism causing septic arthritis.
- In nail pricks *Pseudomonas aeruginosa* is the organism the most common site is the second metatarsophalangeal joint.

GONOCOCCAL ARTHRITIS

The incidence of gonococcal arthritis is less than one percent and it is familiarly known as a three weeks infection. The male to female ratio is 5:1 and the age of predilection is between 20 and 30 years.

It usually results due to lack of treatment for gonorrhea. Forty percent of the cases are monarticular, knee being the most common.

Pathology

Gonococcal arthritis can present as acute, subacute and chronic. The important pathological features are synovitis, effusion, cartilage erosion, and destruction of cartilage.

Clinical Features

Gonococcal arthritis is usually sudden in onset. The patient presents with chills, fever, pain and swelling of the joint. On examination, there is raised temperature and tenderness. There may be history of urethral discharge. The disease may become chronic due to inadequate and improper treatment.

Treatment

The treatment methods consist of local measures like splints, chemotherapy by intravenous penicillin G, and rest to the part, aspiration with a thick bored needle and arthrotomy to clear the joint debris.

SYPHILIS OF JOINTS

The incidence of syphilis of the joints is definitely on the decline due to the early use of antibiotics. Syphilitic arthritis is caused by *Treponema pallidum* and can be classified as follows (Table 2.2).

Investigations

- Wassermann's test is positive.
- *Treponema pallidum* immobilization test is positive.
- Joint fluid aspiration and synovial fluid analysis—for cell, sugar, protein, etc.

Treatment

Antisyphilitic treatment is done but it is often not successful.

Table 2.2: Classification of syphilitic arthritis (for medical readers only)

Congenital	*Acquired*
• **Parrot's syphilitic joint** *Features* – Epiphysitis – Effusion – Separation of epiphysis • **Clutton's joints** *Features* – Symmetrical – Hydrarthrosis – Painless – 8–16 years of age	**Early** • Arthralgia – Secondary stage of syphilis – Nocturnal pain is present – Spasm of muscles • Hydrarthrosis – Serous synovitis – Symmetrical involvement • Gummatous arthritis – Synovial form – Osseous form usually affects the knee, resembles osteoarthritis, painless polyarthritis, etc. • Charcot's joint is a neuropathic joint

NEUROPATHIC JOINTS (Charcot's 1)

This causes extensive destruction of the joint, as it is painless. The following are some of the important causes of neuropathic joints.

- Syringomyelia (25%)
- Tabes dorsalis (4–10%)
- Syphilis
- Rheumatoid arthritis
- Intra-articular steroids
- Traumatic division of sciatic nerve
- Chronic liver disease
- Prolonged administration of drugs like indomethacin.

Sites: Knee, ankle, hip, elbow, shoulder, wrist and intervertebral joints in that order. It is rare before 40 years.

Pathology

The following are the pathological changes seen in the joint—gross destruction of the joint, the capsules are thickened, osteophyte formation is seen, joint cavity is distorted and the loose bodies are present.

Pathological stages (Brailford's stages)
- Stage of hydrarthrosis
- Stage of atrophy
- Stage of hypertrophy.

Clinical Features

In this condition, premonitory signs are rare; onset is usually sudden and unexpected. Gross swelling and lax joint are commonly seen.

In the later stages of the disease, the following features are seen—lax joints, *striking absence of pain*, joint becomes flail and there is a diffuse erythema around the joints.

Radiograph

Gross destruction of the joints is clearly visualized in plain X-rays (Fig. 2.3).

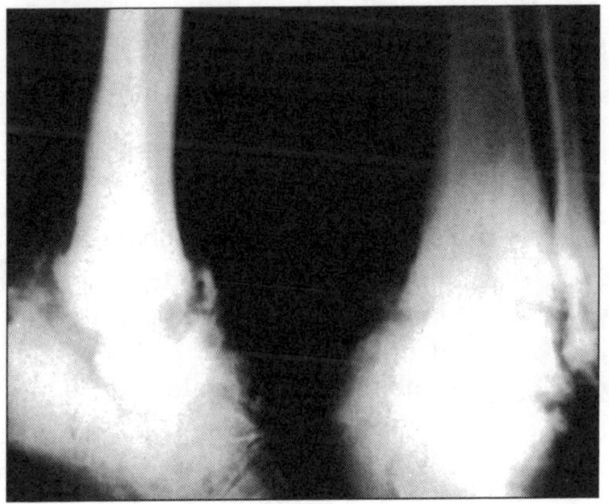

Fig. 2.3: Radiograph showing neuropathic ankle joint

Treatment

The treatment of choice is Charnley's compression arthrodesis but efficient bracing still has a major role to play (Figs 2.4A and B).

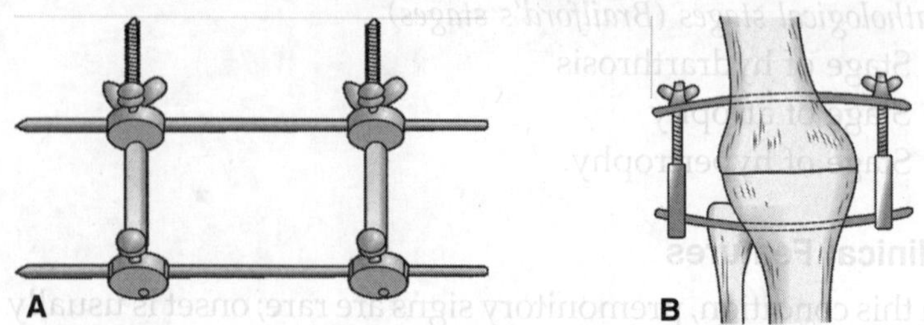

Figs 2.4A and B: (A) Charnley's compression clamp with 2 pins, (B) Charnley's compression arthrodesis

HEMOPHILIC ARTHRITIS (Bleeder's Joints)

Definition

It is a hereditary coagulative disorder characterized by hemorrhages, which is spontaneous and is due to trivial trauma. It is X-linked, carried by female, manifest in male, cause being *prolonged clotting time*. Table 2.3 shows different types of hemophilia.

Incidence is 3–4 per one lakh population.

Severity of factor VIII deficiency and the clinical effects is shown in Table 2.4.

Table 2.3: Types of hemophilia

Hemophilia A	Eighty percent cases due to ↓ factor VIII
Hemophilia B	Fifteen percent due to ↓ factor IX (Christmas disease)
Hemophilia C	Both male and female affected. Autosomal dominant
von Willebrand's disease	Both platelets and factor VIII are deficient.

Table 2.4: Deficiency of factor VIII and its effects

< 1%	Severe bleeding.
< 5%	Gross bleeding with minor trauma.
< 5–25%	Severe bleeding after trauma or surgery.
< 25–50%	Bleeding after excessive trauma or injury.

Pathology

The defective blood interacts with the synovial fluid and causes irritation to the synovial membrane. Due to the proliferation of the macrophages, there is synovial hyper plasia and pannus formation, which ultimately causes destruction of the articular cartilage of the joint (Figs 2.5A to C).

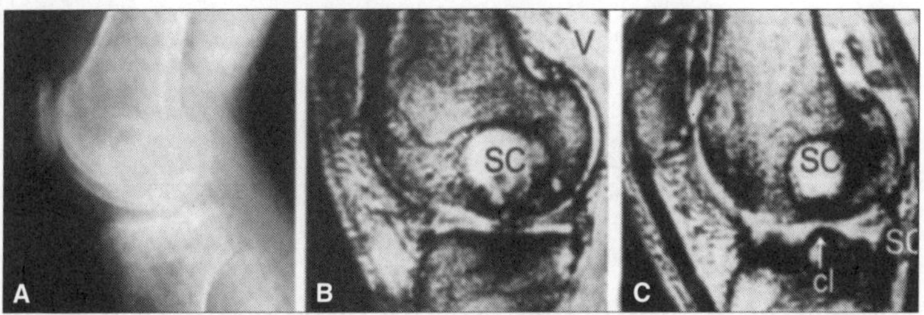

Figs 2.5A to C: Hemophilic arthritis of the knee: (A) Radiograph, (B and C) MRI

Clinical Features

Bleeding is spontaneous and is usually due to trivial trauma. Acute hemarthrosis occurs within hours. The joint is warm, tender and flexion attitude develops. Acute phase lasts for a few weeks. With each attack joint movement decreases, fixed flexion deformity occurs, degenerative arthritis sets in and results in fibrous ankylosis. There is gross muscle atrophy.

Investigations

Plain X-ray

Based on the radiological findings, hemophilia arthritis can be graded into three stages (Table 2.5).

MRI

This gives more information about both the soft tissues and bones of the joints than the conventional radiographs.

Table 2.5: Radiological stages in hemophilia

Early stage	*Intermediate stage*	*End stage*
• Distended synovium • No para-articular skeletal abnormality	• Persistent boggy swelling • Osteoporosis of the epiphysis • Joint interval is normal • Subchondral cysts are present • Squaring of the patella • Intercondylar notch of femur and trochlear notch of ulna widened	• Joint disorganized • Subchondral cysts are large • Fibrous ankylosis is present

Laboratory Tests

The classical feature of this disease is bleeding time is normal, but the clotting time is prolonged. Prothrombin time and other routine laboratory investigations need to be done.

Treatment

This varies according to the stages of the disease.

Acute stage

- For injuries of less than four hours, the patient is treated on OPD basis. Factor VIII is replaced and is discharged home on the same day.
- For injuries more than four hours, factor VIII is replaced; joint is aspirated with a thick bored needle and immobilized with splints.

If resolution	**Recurrence**
Occurs • Patient is mobilized • Caliper wear is suggested	• Factor replacement is done • Immobilization is carried out • Aspiration is done

Late cases: Treated as in-patient, trial aspiration is done, prolonged immobilization, factor VIII is replaced and later mobilization, caliper and splints are recommended.

Chronic Hemarthropathy

For recent contractures: Plaster immobilization, dynamic traction and physiotherapy.

For postsubluxation of tibia: Dynamic traction.

For painful unstable joints: Orthotic splintage.

Surgery is indicated for painful, stiff joints, stiff contractures, and recurrent bleeding into the joint.

Surgical methods: These include synovectomy and internal fixations for fracture nonunion. Supracondylar osteotomy for severe flexion contractures of knee, arthrodesis for severely disorganized joints, total hip replacement for pain in the hip in advanced stages and tendo-Achilles lengthening for tendo-Achilles contractures, etc.

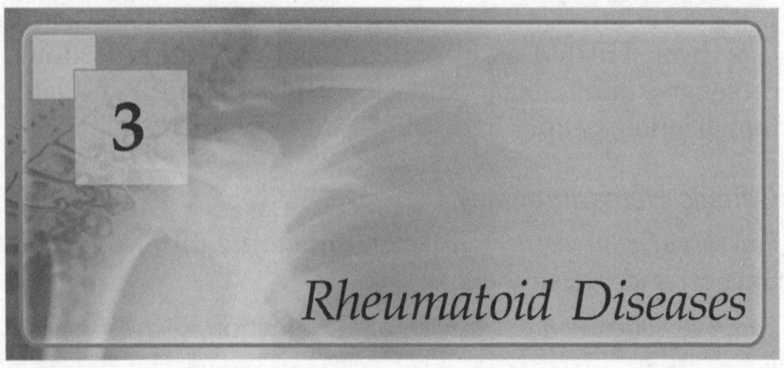

This chapter deals with important inflammatory joint problems in orthopedics

RHEUMATOID ARTHRITIS

Introduction

There is a tendency among the students and most of the clinicians to label all cases of polyarthralgia as rheumatoid arthritis. Though there is no dispute about the fact that the most common cause of polyarthritis is rheumatoid, yet not all cases of polyarthritis is rheumatoid. There is a plethora of conditions with this presentation. Rheumatoid and its variants are infamous in creating diagnostic dilemmas. Difficult to diagnose and difficult to treat, it is indeed a problem which presents a nightmarish experience both to the doctor and the patient.

We are all familiar with the saying regarding rheumatic fever, "It licks the joint but bites the heart." Contrarily, it can be said of rheumatoid arthritis, "It bites the joints, licks all other systems of the body and barks at the treating physicians!"

A chronic scourge, which writes the obituary of the joints, especially those of hands and feet, rheumatoid arthritis, is a problem, which needs to be understood *in toto* to successfully combat it, keep it subdued, and improve the quality of those unfortunate victims afflicted by this malady.

The rheumatic diseases embrace an amazing array of hereditary and acquired disorders with a wide variety of clinical features. As per the present understanding, rheumatic disorders can be classified under three broad headings.

CLASSIFICATION

Diffuse systemic

- Rheumatoid arthritis
- Seronegative spondyloarthritis
- Systemic lupus erythematosus (SLE)
- Polymyositis
- Scleroderma.

Localized articular

- Osteoarthritis
- Crystal-induced arthritis
- Traumatic arthritis.

Nonarticular

- Fibromyalgia
- Low back pain
- Tenosynovitis.

RHEUMATOID ARTHRITIS

Definition

Rheumatoid arthritis is the ***most common*** inflammatory disease of the joints. It is a systemic disease of young and middle-aged adults characterized by proliferative and destructive changes in synovial membrane, periarticular structures, skeletal muscles and perineural sheaths. Eventually, joints are destroyed, fibrosed or ankylosed. *It is a widespread vasculitis of the small arterioles.*

Incidence is 3 percent.

Sex: Eighty percent affected are women; Male: Female ratio is 1:3.

Age: No age is exempt, mean age is 40.

Etiology

The exact cause is unknown, but malfunction of the cellular and humoral arms of the immune system are cited as the probable cause.

Current Hypothesis

An initiating antigen triggers an aberrant response, which becomes self-perpetuating long after the offending antigen has been cleared.

Antigenic Agents

Antigenic agents, which probably act as predisposing factors, are viruses: rubella, Epstein-Barr, etc. genetic (common in people with HLA DR4 60%), psychological stress, allergic factors, endocrine factors and metabolic factors.

Pathogenic Spectrum

Against unknown exciting antigenic agents, rheumatoid factors are elaborated. Rheumatoid factors are synthesized in rheumatoid synovial tissue and are mainly IgM in 70–90 percent of cases. In the remainder 10–30 percent, it could be IgG, IgA or IgE. This rheumatoid factor along with IgG triggers off a compliment cascade. The WBCs engulf this immune complex and elaborate lysosomes. Neutrophils release procollagenase, which is converted into an active collagenase by the synovial fluid. This splits the collagen of the articular cartilage. The neutral proteases complete the degradation of the collagen fibrils (Fig. 3.1).

Pathology

As explained earlier, due to the synthesis of autoantibodies, against unknown antigenic agents in the synovium, primary synovitis sets in (Fig. 3.2). This primary synovitis gives rise to pannus, which in turn forms the villus. This villus migrates towards the joint causing its destruction and ankylosis, fibrous in the early stages followed by bony ankylosis in the late stages.

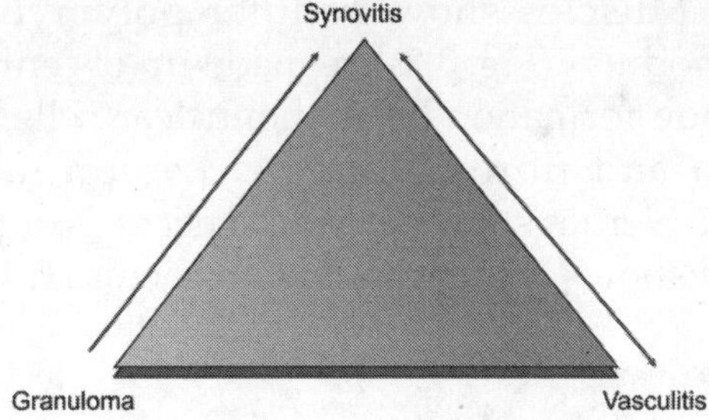

Fig. 3.1: Rheumatoid arthritis = Synovitis + vasculitis + granuloma

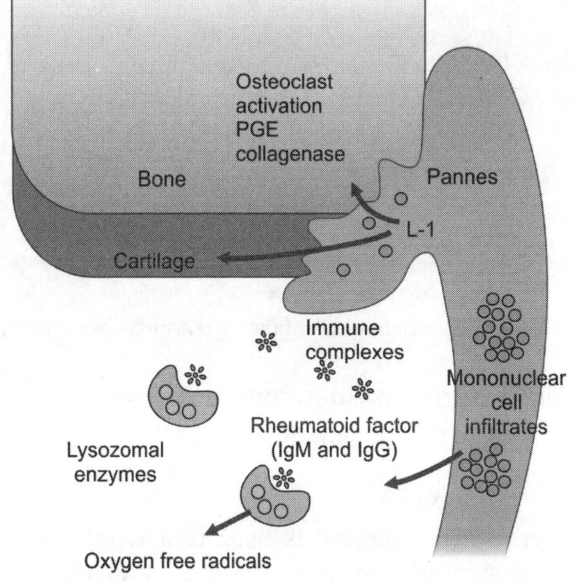

Fig. 3.2: Pathogenesis in rheumatoid arthritis

Microscopy

It reveals rheumatoid units, which are an area of fibrinoid necrosis surrounded by fibroblasts, arranged radially and it is surrounded by a fibrous capsule. This rheumatoid unit is found in the muscle, vessels, nerves, synovium, etc. Vasculitis is widespread, and commonly affects the arterioles. Muscles show nodular polymyositis. Subcutaneous nodules (Fig. 3.3) are made-up of central necrotic area, palisade formation by mononuclear cells, round cell infiltration and fibrous capsule. Lymph nodes show hyperplasia. Nerves show perineural necrosis or fibrosis and heart rarely shows changes unlike in rheumatic fever.

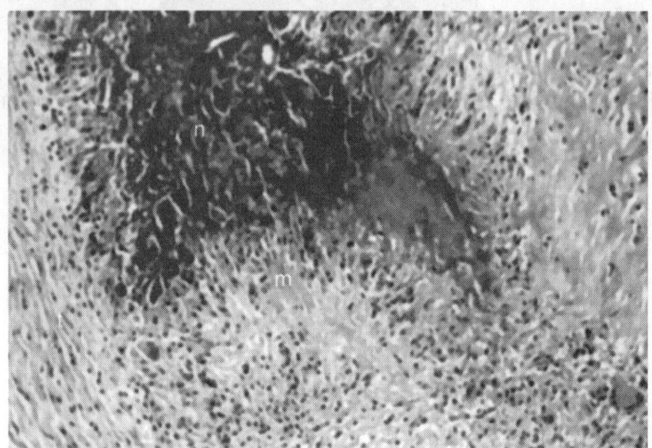

Fig. 3.3: Microscopic features of rheumatoid arthritis subcutaneous nodule

Clinical Features in Rheumatoid Arthritis

Rheumatoid arthritis usually presents in three forms:

Classical Presentation

In this group, the patient is usually a woman in her mid-30s. Pain, swelling, stiffness of the small joints of hands and feet are the common presenting complaints. The patient also gives history of weight loss, lethargy and depression. Joint swelling could be symmetrical and the patient presents with deformities of bones and joints in the late stages. *The patient gives history of remissions and exacerbation of symptoms with seasonal variations.* This is a very classical complaint in the absence of which diagnosis of rheumatoid arthritis should be carefully made. Symptoms fluctuate from day to day.

Recent diagnostic criteria for rheumatoid arthritis

According to the American College of Rheumatology in 1987 revised criteria, at least 4 out of 7 criteria should be fulfilled to make a diagnosis of rheumatoid arthritis.

- Morning stiffness for minimum one hour everyday, at least for six weeks.
- Arthritis or swelling of three or more joints for > 6 weeks.
- Arthritis or swelling of hand joints (wrist, metacarpal) for more than 6 weeks.
- Symmetrical swelling (arthritis of same joint areas) more than 6 weeks.
- Serum rheumatoid factor present.
- Radiographic features of RA.
- Rheumatoid nodules.

Other Presentations

This consists of palindromic presentation involving one or two joints, systemic presentation—usually seen in middle-aged men presenting with pleurisy, pericarditis, etc. It mimics malignancy. It may present as polymyalgia particularly in elderly patients. It may present as monoarthritic swelling. Sometimes the presentation may be very explosive unlike the usual chronic presentation.

Extra-articular Features

Two or more features are present in 75 percent of the cases. Rheumatoid factor is invariably present and indicates a bad prognosis.

- Subcutaneous nodules are present in 25 percent of the cases. It is seen over the elbow, sacrum and occiput. Nodules may also be present in lungs, eye, hearts, etc. When present over flexor tendon, it may cause trigger finger.
- Widespread vasculitis.
- Blood abnormalities commonly encountered in rheumatoid arthritis are chronic anemia, iron deficiency anemia, vitamin B_{12} and folate deficiency, leukocytopenia, thrombocytosis and marrow hypoplasia.

- Osteoporosis could be generalized or localized in bones around the joints.
- Eye changes seen in rheumatoid arthritis are keratoconjunctivitis sicca or Sjögren's syndrome, episcleritis (common), scleritis (serious problem), secondary glaucoma and scleromalacia perforans.
- Lung affections in rheumatoid arthritis are pleurisy, pleural effusion, Kaplan's syndrome (RA + pneumoconiosis involving the upper lobes) and fibrosing alveolitis in 2 percent.
- Heart affections in rheumatoid arthritis are pericardial friction (10%), pericardial effusion (30%), arrhythmias and heart block.
- Neuromuscular system involvement includes carpal tunnel syndrome, mononeuritis multiplex, muscle wasting, subluxation of C1 and C2, etc.
- Reticuloendothelial system affections include splenomegaly (5%), Felty's syndrome in 1% (RA+ splenomegaly + Neutropenia), generalized lymphadenopathy and painless pitting edema of the feet and ankles.

ORTHOPEDIC DEFORMITIES IN RHEUMATOID ARTHRITIS

Rheumatoid arthritis can affect any joint in the body. *It involves the peripheral joints more often and very rarely affects the larger joints*. Of particular importance are the affection of the temporomandibular joint and atlantoaxial joint, which can prove lethal due to the cord compression. Figure 3.4 shows frequency of involvement of various joints in rheumatoid arthritis.

Quick Facts

Joints involved in rheumatoid arthritis

- Metacarpophalangeal and interphalangeal joints of the hand.
- Shoulder elbow and wrists.
- Hip, knee and ankle.

Others: Temporomandibular joint, atlantoaxial joints and facet joints of the cervical spine.

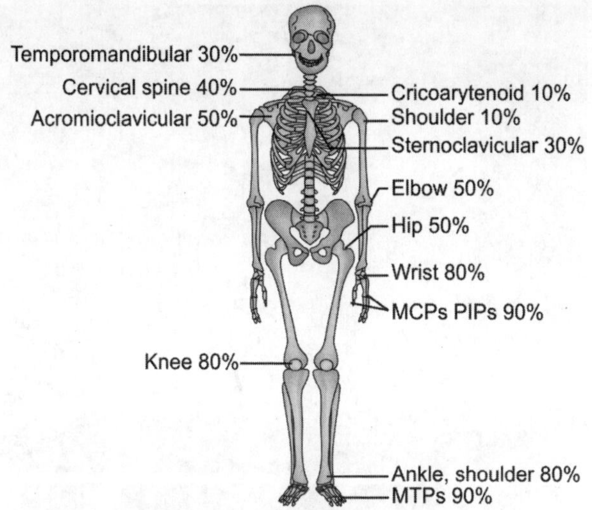

Fig. 3.4: Frequency of involvement of different joint sites in established RA

Orthopedic Deformities of the Hand (Rheumatoid hand)

Orthopedic deformities of the hand (rheumatoid hand) the following are some of the very common deformities seen in the hand (Figs 3.5A to C).

- *Symmetrical peripheral joint swelling* of metacarpophalangeal and interphalangeal joints (Fig. 3.5A).
- *Ulnar deviation* of the hand is due to rupture of the collateral ligaments at the metacarpophalangeal joints, which enables the extensor tendons to slip from their grooves towards the ulnar side (Figs 3.6A and B).
- *Boutonniere's deformity* is due to the rupture of central extensor expansion of the fingers resulting in flexion at the PIP joint (Fig. 3.5C).
- *Swan neck deformity* is due to the rupture of the volar plate of the PIP joints, which enables the tendons to slip towards the dorsal side. This is also known as *intrinsic plus deformity*. Here there is hyperextension of the PIP joint and flexion of the DIP joints.

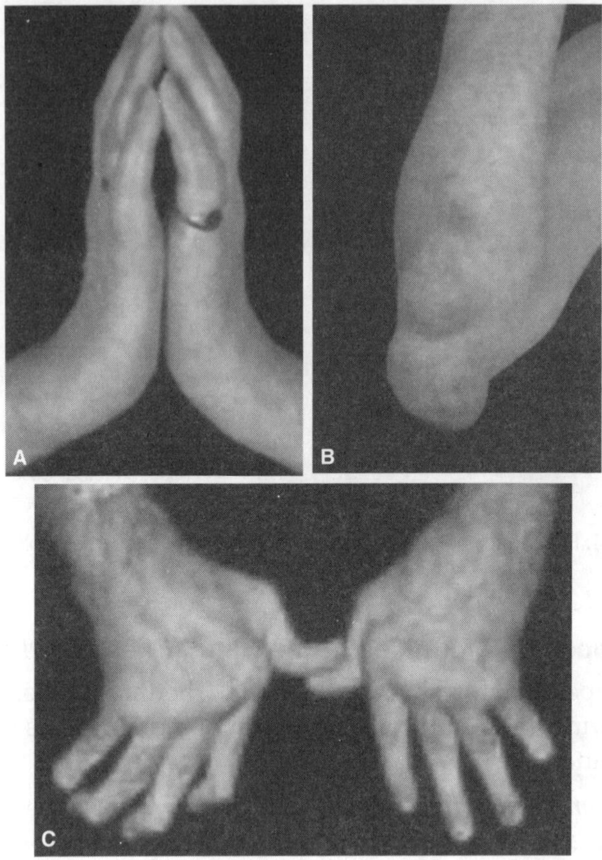

Figs 3.5A to C: Rheumatic features of the hand and the elbow (clinical photo)

- *Trigger fingers and trigger thumb are* due to nodules over the tendons.
- Z-deformity of the thumb.
- Subluxation and dislocation of metacarpophalangeal joints.

Rheumatoid Foot

It affects the forefoot, midfoot and hindfoot. In the forefoot, the patient may develop hallux valgus deformity of the great

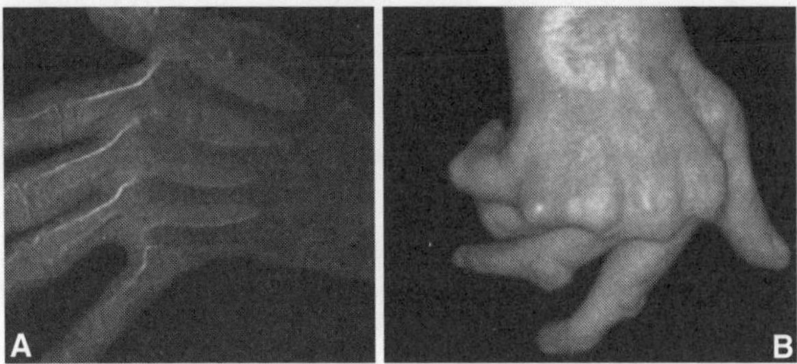

Figs 3.6A and B: Rheumatoid hand (clinical photo)

toe, claw toes, callosity over the dorsum and the sole, widening of the forefoot, etc. The heel may show valgus deformity.

Ninety percent of patients with rheumatoid arthritis of long-standing duration have foot deformities. Forefoot is more commonly affected than the hind foot (Also see box).

Vital facts: About foot deformities in rheumatoid arthritis:

- Callosity under PIP joint
- Plantar callosity
- Atrophy of plantar metatarsal fat pad
- Prominent metatarsal head
- Excessive plantar tilt of metatarsals
- Claw toes
- Hammer toes
- Rheumatoid nodules
- Calcaneal erosions
- Achilles tendinitis
- Flattening of longitudinal arch
- Bunion
- Hallux valgus
- Overriding of second and third toes
- Splaying of forefoot due to divergent metatarsals.

Other Joints

In the knee initially there is a gross soft tissue swelling due to synovitis; and in the later stages, the patient may develop fibrous ankylosis or bony ankylosis due to widespread destruction of the articular cartilage by the pannus. Similarly, other major joints of the body like the hip, ankle, shoulder, and elbow could be involved.

Do you know the frequency of joint involvement in rheumatoid arthritis? (Fig. 3.4)

- MCP/MTP/PIP joints — 90 percent
- Knee, ankle and wrist — 80 percent
- Shoulder — 60 percent
- Hip, elbow, acromion — 50 percent
- Cervical spine — 40 percent
- Temporomandibular and sternomastoid joints — 30 percent
- Cricoarytenoid joint — 10 percent

Note: Characteristically distal interphalangeal joint and sacroiliac joint are not involved in rheumatoid arthritis.

Investigation

Laboratory

Hb percentage is low and shows normochromic, hypochromic anemia. WBCs are decreased or normal, there are increased lymphocytes and the ESR is raised.

Serological Tests

Basis: Rheumatoid patient's serum contains RA factor, which in the presence of γ-globulin agglutinates certain strains of streptococci sensitized by sheep cells and latex particles.

- *Latex fixation test:* Unknown serum + 7-globulin latex suspension

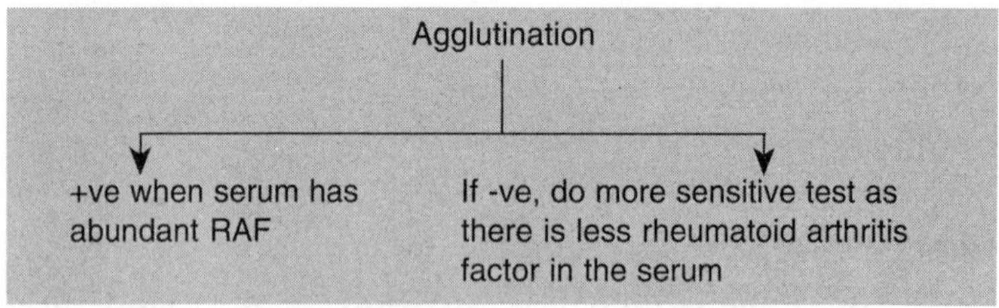

- *Inhibition test:* This test uses the characteristics of euglobulin from unknown serum. Euglobulin from normal serum neutralizes the rheumatoid factor thereby inhibiting agglutination.

Euglobulin from rheumatoid serum has no effect on the rheumatoid factor and agglutination occurs. *This is the most sensitive test*. Positive even when rheumatoid arthritis factor is present in minute amounts.

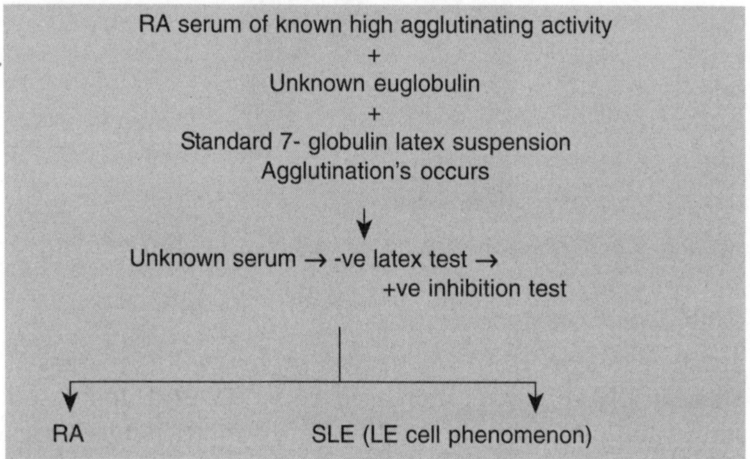

Remember

RA factor is found in

- 75 percent of rheumatoid arthritis cases
- 10 percent in healthy elderly people
- 10 percent in malaria, etc.

Radiological Features of Rheumatoid Arthritis (Fig. 3.7)

- Soft tissue swelling.
- Juxta-articular osteoporosis.
- Erosion of joint margins.
- Joint spaces are decreased.
- Deformities.
- Atlantoaxial subluxation.
- Subchondral erosions and cyst formation.
- Fibrous and bony ankylosis develops in the late stages.

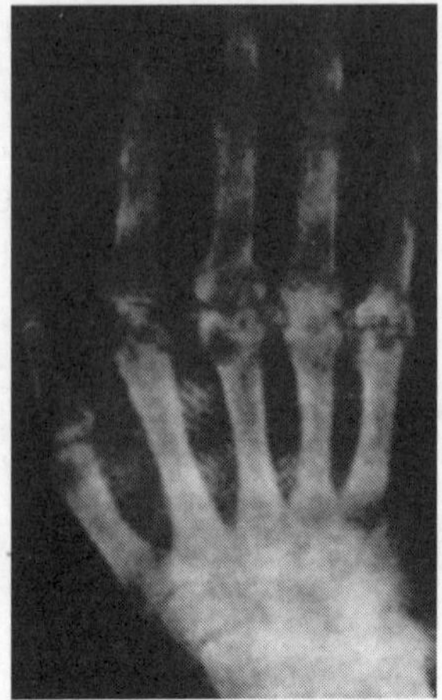

Fig. 3.7: Radiograph showing features of rheumatoid arthritis

Other Common Abnormalities

These include increased C-reactive protein (CRP), increased alkaline phosphatase, increased platelets, and decreased serum albumin. Citrulline antibody is present in most cases of early rheumatoid arthritis. Antinuclear antibody (ANA) is also frequently raised in patients with rheumatoid arthritis.

Synovial Fluid Analysis

This is not performed routinely for diagnostic purposes but performed to exclude other causes of inflammation such as infection.

Synovial fluid in RA is typically yellow, watery and turbid due to high WBC and has low sugar content.

MRI

This gives valuable information about the various soft tissue damages in rheumatoid with far more greater accuracy (Fig. 3.8).

Differential Diagnosis

Differential diagnosis of rheumatoid arthritis with various other conditions is shown in Table 3.1. However, for the

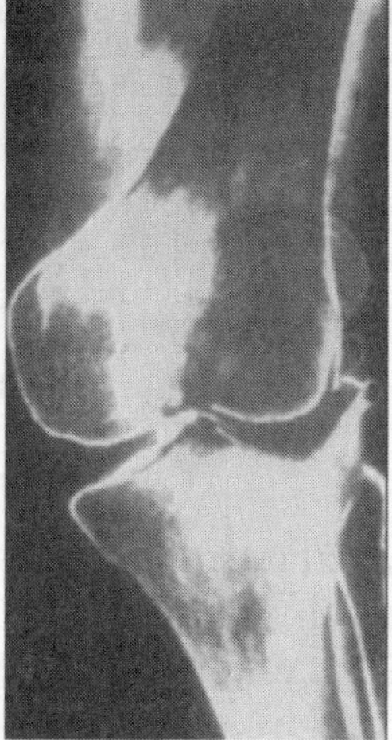

Fig. 3.8: MRI rheumatoid knee

differential diagnosis of rheumatoid arthritis with the all-important osteoarthritis (Table 3.2).

Quick facts of rheumatoid arthritis

- Most common chronic inflammatory disorder.
- 80 percent in women.
- Exact cause is not known.
- Rheumatoid unit is present.
- History of remissions and exacerbations present.
- Symmetrical peripheral joint involvement.
- Rheumatoid arthritis factor is +ve in 70 percent.
- Inhibition test is most sensitive.
- Extra-articular features are seen in 75 percent.

Management

Aims of Treatment

- To keep inflammatory process at a minimum, thereby, preserving joint motion, maintaining healthy muscles and preventing secondary joint stiffness and deformity (Fig. 3.9).
- To keep constitutional symptoms at a minimum.
- The possible deformities are anticipated and prevented by appropriate splinting.

Table 3.1: Differential diagnosis of rheumatoid arthritis

Early disease	*Established disease*
Common • Viral arthropathy • Polymyalgia • Infection • Prodrome of hepatitis • Hypoparathyroidism	**Common** • Psoriatic arthritis • Erosive osteoarthritis • Chronic pyrophosphate disease • Chronic tophaceous gout • SLE • Reiter's syndrome • Ankylosing spondylitis
Rare • Sarcoidosis • Acute leukemia • Coeliac disease • Eosinophilic fasciitis	**Rare** • Amyloid arthropathy • Multicentric reticulohistio-cytosis

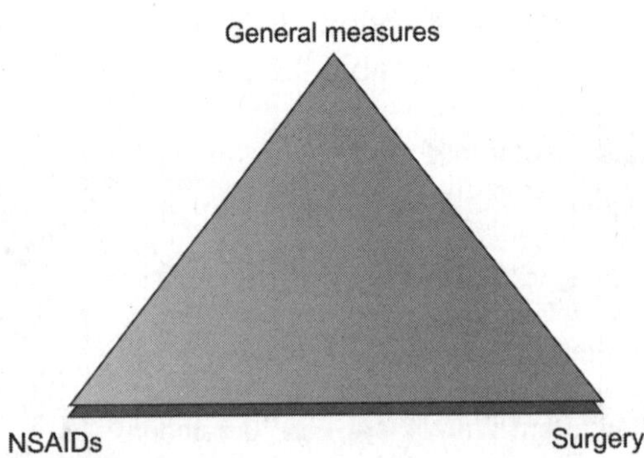

Fig. 3.9: Treatment triad for rheumatoid arthritis

- Finally, surgical measures to correct the deformities, eliminate pain and provide stability are undertaken.

General Measures

It aims at improving the general condition of the patient and to keep the joints properly splinted in functional position to guard against the ensuing ankylosis.

Table 3.2: Differences between rheumatoid arthritis and osteoarthritis

Rheumatoid arthritis	*Osteoarthritis*
• It is an autoimmune disease and often strikes in the prime of life.	• It is an age-related disease due to wear and tear of the cartilage.
• It is usually seen between the ages of 25 and 50 years of age but can also occur in children and infancy.	• It usually affects people after 40 years of age.
• It affects joints on both sides of the body and has a bilateral presentation.	• It usually affects isolated joints, or joints on only one side of the body at first.
• It causes redness, warmth and swelling of the joints.	• It usually does not cause redness and warmth of the joints.
• It affects many joints usually small joints of the hands and feet, and may affect the elbow, shoulders, wrist, hip, knee and ankles.	• It most commonly affects weightbearing joints or joints that are overused (e.g. knees and hip).
• It can affect the entire system, with general feeling of sickness and fatigue, as well as weight loss.	• Discomfort is usually related to the affected joint.
	• Brief morning stiffness.
• There is history of prolonged morning stiffness.	• It rarely causes fatigue.
• It causes major fatigue.	

- Rest in bed.
- Good diet, rich in proteins and minerals.
- Transfusion and hematinics to correct the anemia.
- Hormones combination of estrogen and androgen to improve the bone stock.
- Removal of infective foci.

Splinting in the functional position helps in the event that ankylosis ensues. The splint is removed daily. Hot packs are given or the patient is placed in Hubbard tank at (92.6–102°F) and the joints are put into full range of motion.

While the joints are immobilized, muscle-setting exercises are advocated. After removal of the splints, resistance exercises are begun.

Splints

These are known to serve three main functions:

- Rest and relief of pain (*rest splints*).
- Prevention and correction of deformity (*corrective splints*).
- Fixation of damaged joint in a good functional position (*fixation splints*).

Drug Therapy

Three classes of drugs are used regularly

- Analgesics
- Anti-inflammatory drugs
- Disease modifying drugs.

Steroids especially intra-articular injections have an important role.

No treatment is ideal and it is important to assess the patient's response so that the most effective regimen is adopted.

Commonly used methods of assessment include; duration of early morning stiffness, number of tender swollen joints. Functional assessment, questionnaires, ESR, radiographs, etc.

First Line of Drugs: NSAIDs

These are aspirin/ibuprofen/ketoprofen/diclofenac sodium/naproxen/piroxicam, etc. They are the major pharmaceutical agents for pain relief in rheumatic diseases. About 20 percent of patients admitted to the hospital are taking NSAIDs. Though useful, they have significant side effects. Steroids are useful during flare ups.

Aspirin is the *drug of first choice;* but because of its undesirable side effects, other NSAIDs are chosen. However, since the latter are more expensive, aspirin remains the first choice drug.

Mechanism of action of NSAIDs: They have an inhibitory action on the following pain-mediating agents:

- Prostaglandin synthesis
- Leukotriene synthesis
- Lymphocyte activation
- Oxygen radical generation
- Cytokine production, etc.

Practical Prescribing of NSAIDs: There is no ideal NSAID. It is important to become familiar with a few of these drugs and to find the most appropriate NSAID for one particular patient. *If possible, NSAIDs should be prescribed twice-daily regimen, with a flexible dose to cover the main period of pain.* Initially, clinicians should prescribe NSAIDs with which they are familiar and not necessarily the latest drug.

Only one NSAID should be prescribed at one time and if the patient has not responded to an adequate dose within 2–3 weeks, an alternative NSAID should be given.

It is important to justify the use of NSAID, both in the short- and long-term. Other methods of pain relief should always be considered, such as exercises, heat and cold hydrotherapy.

Quick facts of NSAIDs

- Drugs of first choice
- Aspirin remains as the first choice
- There are no ideal NSAIDs
- Prescribe NSAID with which clinician is familiar
- Ideal is twice daily regimen
- Only one NSAID at a time
- To be tried for a minimum of 2–3 weeks
- NSAIDs provide only symptomatic relief.

NSAIDs provide only symptomatic relief. Most patients require daily treatment. These drugs probably do not have any influence on the disease process and may, therefore, be regarded as a background therapy with a variable daily dose according to symptoms.

Second Line of Drugs

Second line of drugs are used only if an adequate trial of first line drugs have failed to relieve symptoms satisfactorily or if there is radiological evidence of progressive disease. Second line drugs are alternatively known as *disease modifying antirheumatic drugs (DMARD)* and are slow acting drugs. It would seem that they have influence on the underlying disease process, and may take several weeks or months to exert this effect.

To get maximum benefit, second line drug therapy should be continued for *at least 6 months;* and in order to sustain the benefit, it needs to be continued indefinitely. They are all toxic.

When second line therapy is introduced, *symptomatic NSAIDs need to be continued in parallel.* If the response to the second line drug is good, the dose of NSAID can be reduced.

Commonly prescribed drugs include:

- Injectable gold and oral gold (sodium aurothiomalate). This is no longer preferred.
- Penicillamine
- Sulphasalazine
- Antimalarial drugs (e.g. chloroquine)
- Dapsone and levamisole.

The choice of the drug to be given first will depend on the experience of the doctor and on the facilities available for monitoring. There is little evidence to suggest which drug should be prescribed first.

If after 6 months of adequate therapy, no response has been observed, an alternative drug may be tried.

At the end of a year of the treatment, 65 percent would have improved, 35 percent will have had to stop therapy because of toxicity or lack of therapeutic effect.

Currently, gold satts are on the decline due to their side effects. Methotrexate has now emerged as the drug of choice due to its higher efficacy. Early institution and escalation of MTX to its maximum tolerable dose is the latest mantra.

Antimalarial Drugs

They do not require intensive blood monitoring and if these facilities are limited, chloroquine or hydroxy chloroquine can be particularly used.

Other agents known to have second line drug effect include levamisole and dapsone. Levamisole is not freely available in some countries and its toxicity seems to be greater than that of gold and penicillamine. Dapsone has a high toxicity.

Indications of second line drugs: The ideal patient for a second line drug is one who has active synovitis with generalized inflammation in many joints, who is taking the recommended dose of the NSAID which is not producing relief of symptoms.

Quick facts of second line drugs

- Used only if first line fails.
- Known as DMARD.
- To be continued for at least 6 months.
- Parallel NSAID is to be used.
- Choice of drugs is based on clinicians' experience.
- Antimalarial drugs are used if proper blood monitoring is not available.
- All drugs are toxic.

Third Line of Drugs

Azathioprim, cyclophosphamide and chlorambucil can exert a second line effect inpatients with rheumatoid arthritis. However, these drugs are considered under third line drugs because in addition to the toxicity, which may arise acutely during their use, *there is also anxiety about late toxicity*. This late toxicity, which may occur after prolonged therapy, is an additional hazard for patients who are suffering from what is essentially a non-fatal condition. These drugs have, therefore, to be treated with respect though in selected cases they may be of benefit.

Corticosteroids: Cyclosporine has been tried inpatients with rheumatoid arthritis. The fact that it does not affect WBC is a theoretical advantage inpatients with Felty's syndrome. Anxieties about longterm nephrotoxicity limit the use of cyclosporine to research programes.

Newer Drugs for Rheumatoid Arthritis

- Tumor Necrosis Factor (INF α-blockers)

For example

a. Etanarcept (25 mg/subcutaneous, twice a week)
b. Infliximab (2 mg/kg at 0, 6, 8 and weekly. IV infusions combined with oral methotrexate).
c. Interleukin-1-receptor antagonist (IL-IRA) Dose—100 mg/day by subcutaneous injection.

Indications

Failure of at least two standard DMARD drugs one of which is always methotrexate despite adequate trials (i.e. 6 months).

- Leflunomide (immunomodulatory drug)
  Indicated dose is 100 mg/day for 3 days then 20 mg/day.

Local Steroids

Role of local corticosteroid treatment is considered when the rheumatoid arthritis affects one or two joints. It is also indicated in tendinitis, capsular or ligament involvement, carpal tunnel and compression syndromes. It is given weekly in acute cases and three monthly in chronic. *If two injections are ineffective, the treatment is discontinued.*

Surgical Procedures in Rheumatology

Aim of surgery in rheumatoid arthritis is to:

- Relieve pain.
- Correct the deformity of the joints.
- Reduce joint instability.
- Improve the range of movements of the joints.

Surgical advice should be sought only when the disease is *clearly progressive and conservative measures are failing*, but before the patient starts to lose a significant amount of bone stock. If surgery is delayed, more bone is lost, the soft tissue deteriorates and the deformity increases.

Preoperative Considerations

Before surgery for rheumatoid disease, a number of specific points should be checked. Related conditions such as diabetes, hypertension and anemia should be adequately treated and:

- Steroid dosage should be reduced.
- There should be no active infection.
- A radiograph of the cervical spine should be obtained to exclude instability.

Modus operandi of surgical procedures in rheumatoid arthritis

Synovectomy	• Failed chemotherapy • Joint destruction should be minimal • Useful in knee/ankle
Osteotomy	• Less than 60 years of age • When joint is partially damaged • Commonly done at hip (Intertrochanteric osteotomy and abduction osteotomy)
Arthrodesis	• Long-term relief • Reserved for peripheral joints where arthroplasty results in pain • Causes secondary osteoarthritis in bigger joints
Arthroplasty	• Advanced stages in hip and knee

Surgical Methods

Synovectomy

It may be indicated in patients with rheumatoid arthritis if joint destruction is minimal and if the main cause of pain and swelling is synovitis, which is resistant to medication and physiotherapy. Synovectomy is usually carried out over the knee and ankle, in the elbow with radial head excision if necessary. In the wrist, dorsal synovectomy and resection of the distal end of the ulna can prevent attrition and rupture of extensor tendons. *Synovectomy has to be virtually complete to avoid regrowth with recurrence of symptoms.*

Osteotomy

This should be considered in patients under the age of 60 years with osteoarthritis of the hip or knee due to rheumatoid arthritis. *Osteotomy has the advantage of relieving pain without sacrificing the joint surfaces, which have only been partially damaged.*

At the hip, intertrochanteric osteotomy, which contains the femoral head within the acetabulum, is preferred. At the knee, abduction osteotomy is preferred.

Arthrodesis

Arthrodesis of the joint gives excellent long-term pain relief. Nevertheless, the stress may cause secondary OA in the adjacent joints unless they are able to compensate for the loss of movement. Lack of movement after fusion of the wrist can be absorbed at the elbow and shoulder without significant functional impairment, but fusion of the hip puts considerable strain on the spine and the knee.

Arthrodesis, therefore, tends to be preserved for peripheral joints, such as the wrist, ankle, and IP joints of the hands and feet where the functional loss is less disabling and arthroplasty is less reliable.

Arthroplasties

Arthroplasties of the hip, knee (Figs 3.10A and B), ankle, shoulder, elbow, wrist, and hand is indicated in advanced diseases causing severe pain and incapacitating disability due to stiffness and instability.

Self-management Techniques for Rheumatoid and other Forms of Arthritis

Self-management is the most important aspect of the treatment of rheumatoid and other forms of arthritis. People practicing self-management techniques tend to experience less pain and are more active than those who do not practice self-management. In this management, the patient is made aware of the disease and the rationale behind the treatment. They are made to realize that the success of the treatment is their ultimate responsibility.

Ten Self-help Techniques

1. *Positive mental attitude*: The patient is told to focus on things other than pain and their own body. They are encouraged to think positively (Fig. 3.11A).
2. *Regular medication*: The patient is told the value of regular and correct medication (Fig. 3.11B).
3. *Regular exercises*: The patient should follow a regular and appropriate exercise program, most suited for them (Fig. 3.11C).
4. *Use of joints*: The patient is told the value of correct posture and the methods of using the joints wisely to reduce stress on the painful joints (Fig. 3.11D).
5. *Energy conservation*: Patients are instructed to listen to the body's "inner signals" for rest. Slowing down and avoiding too many activities reduces the stress on the joints.

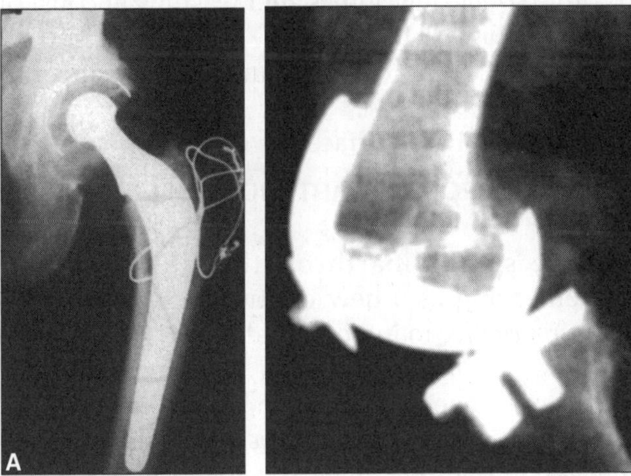

Figs 3.10A and B: Radiographs showing: (A) Total hip replacement, (B) Total knee replacement for rheumatoid arthritis of the hip and knee

6. *Assistive devices*: Devices like splints, braces and walking sticks can help stabilize the joints, provide strength and reduce pain and inflammation (Fig. 3.11F).
7. *Adequate sleep*: A good adequate sleep provides rest to the ailing joints and reduces the pain and swelling (Fig. 3.11G).
8. *Massage*: A good moderate massage brings warmth and relieves pain due to arthritis (Fig. 3.11H).
9. *Relaxation techniques*: Relaxation techniques like yoga, meditation, etc. help to relax the muscles, mind and controls respiration, heart rate, blood pressure. This helps in the control of pain (Fig. 3.11I).
10. *Modification in the daily activities*
    - Using Western toilets (Fig. 3.11J)
    - Bath aids and railings
    - Long handle broomstick and mop to clean the floors (Fig. 3.11E)
    - Use of walking sticks while walking, climbing, etc.
    - High chairs
    - Avoid squatting on the ground for food, etc. Use of dining table and chairs are recommended
    - To avoid squeezing clothes after washing and just rinse them dry (Fig. 3.11J)
    - To avoid walking on hard and uneven and rough surfaces
    - To sleep on a hard surface.

SERONEGATIVE SPONDYLOARTHROPATHIES

Introduction

Seronegative spondyloarthropathies (SSA) group is gradually emerging as a new entity. These disorders are labeled as *seronegative* to indicate that they have in common the *absence of the rheumatoid factor*. The term spondylo-arthropathies is used because in many cases there is involvement of the *spine and sacroiliac joints*. Hence, SSA can be defined as an *acute or chronic condition with characteristic involvement of axial joints, absence of RA factor and HLA abnormality*.

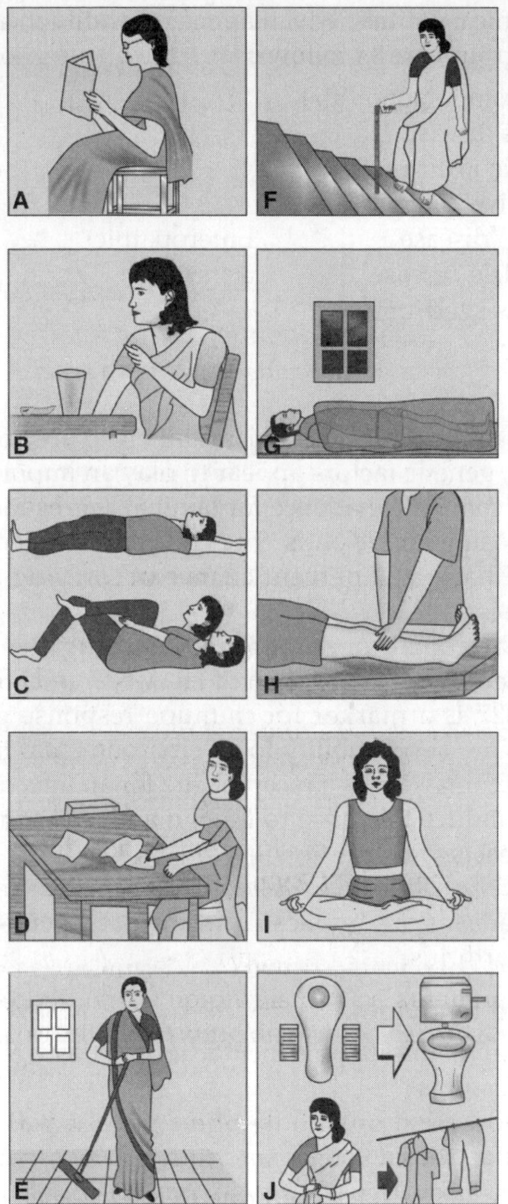

Figs 3.11A to J: Self-management techniques in the treatment of rheumatoid arthritis

The clinical entities, which appear to justify inclusions in the SSA group, are as follows:

- Ankylosing spondylitis
- Reiter's disease
- Psoriatic arthritis
- Ulcerative colitis
- Crohn's disease } Enteropathic arthritis
- Whipple's disease }
- Behçet's syndrome

Etiology

The exact pathogenic mechanisms involved are not known. However, genetic factors appear to play an important role. The most complete evidence for familial aggregation is that for ankylosing spondylitis. The children of a person with HLA-B27 have a 50 percent chance of carrying the same antigen.

There are some postulations regarding the possible mechanism for the association of HLA-B27 and SSA.

- HLA-B27 is a marker for immune response gene that determines susceptibility to an environmental trigger.
- HLA-B27 may act as a receptor site for an infective agent.
- It may induce tolerance to foreign antigen with which it cross-reacts.

Salmonella, Shigella, Chlamydia, Yersinia and other microorganisms are implicated in the pathogenesis of this group of arthritis.

Signs and Symptoms

The clinical manifestations include *articular* as well as *extra-articular* features.

Articular Features

These include low back pain due to progressive sacroiliitis and spondylitis. The patient complains of morning stiffness and decreasing lumbar lordosis.

Diffuse swelling of fingers and toes may occur due to small joint synovitis and tenosynovitis. The manifestation is referred to as *sausage digit.* Enthesopathy, i.e. pain at the site of insertion of ligaments and tendons can occur at Achilles tendon, plantar fascia and ischial tuberosities.

Extra-articular Features

These features include skin lesions such as *psoriasis, pitting of nails*, and penile ulcers, eye lesions like conjunctivitis, bowel disorders and genitourinary disturbances such as *dysuria* and *urethral discharge.*

Diagnosis

Radiological Diagnosis

Radiological diagnosis *forms one of the proven diagnostic techniques in diagnosing SSA.* Radiological study of the affected joints will show *punched out areas* exceeding deep into the subchondral bone.

CAT Scan

CAT scan is also a very useful method that helps in the diagnosis. *It is indicated when plain X-rays are normal.* Early changes of sclerosis and bone erosion, which are not visible on a plain X-ray, can be clearly demonstrated on CAT scan.

HLA-B27

HLA-B27 shows a strong association with SSA. Its presence adds weight to the diagnosis of these conditions. The frequency of its occurrence with SSA ranges between 16 and 100 percent. In ankylosing spondylitis, the frequency of its occurrence is as high as 85–90 percent, while in Behçet's syndrome it is as low as 16 percent. *In all patients of SSA, the RA factor is uniformly negative.*

One of the diagnostic pitfalls encountered is a mistaken diagnosis of RA. Hence, at the very outset, it is essential to differentiate between these two conditions (Table 3.3).

Table 3.3: Difference between SSA and RA

	SSA	*RA*
Age	Young usually less than 40 years	Any age group
Sex	Predominantly Male	Predominantly females
Symmetry	Usually asymmetrical	Usually symmetrical
Number of joints involved	Oligoarticular	Polyarticular
Spine involvement	Common	Only cervical spine
Enthesopathy	Typical	Not a feature
RA factor	Typically –ve	Typically +ve
HLA-B27	+ ve in high Percentage	–ve in normal population

ANKYLOSING SPONDYLITIS (Syn: Marie-Strumpell Disease)

Definition

This is a chronic progressive inflammatory disease of the sacroiliac joints and the axial skeleton.

Causes

Causes are unknown. It is found to be strongly associated with HLA-B27 genetic marker (about 85 percent).

The infective triggers are certain gram-negative organisms more so *Klebsiella*.

Age/sex Common in young male adults (M : F = 10:1).

Pathology

The initial inflammation of the joints is followed by synovitis, arthritis, and cartilage destruction, fibrous and later bony ankylosis. The joints commonly affected are SI joints, spine, hip, and knee and manubrium sterni.

Clinical Features

The patient usually complains of early morning stiffness and pain in the back. On examination patient has a stiff spine.

Tests for sacroiliac joint involvement are positive (Figs 3.12 to 3.14). Cervical spine involvement is tested by asking the patient to touch the wall with the back of the head without raising his or her chin (Fleche's test). If the chest expansion is less than 5 cm, involvement of thoracic spine is suspected (Fig. 3.15). Gradually, a progressive kyphotic deformity of the entire spine develops (Fig. 3.16).

Diagnostic criteria for ankylosing spondylitis

- Insidious onset
- Age < 40 years
- Persistence for > 3 months
- Morning stiffness
- Improvement with exercise

Extra-articular Manifestations

These include acute iritis (25%), pericarditis, aortic incompetence, subluxation of atlantoaxial joints, apical lobe fibrosis, generalized osteoporosis, etc.

Differential Diagnosis

For differential diagnosis of various types of SSA, see Table 3.4. For differences between ankylosing spondylitis and backache due to other causes, see Table 3.5.

Investigations

Radiographs of SI joint show haziness, subchondral erosions, sclerosis (Fig. 3.17A) widening of SI joint, etc.

Radiographs of spine show squaring of vertebra, loss of lumbar lordosis, calcification of anterior longitudinal ligament bridging osteophytes, bamboo spine (Fig. 3.17B), etc.

Other investigations: This consists of CT scan, MRI, and bone scan, etc.

Laboratory investigations HLA-B27 is raised in 95 percent, raised ESR is seen in 50 percent and serum IgA is significantly increased.

Treatment

- *General measures:* This is extremely important and consists of the following measures:

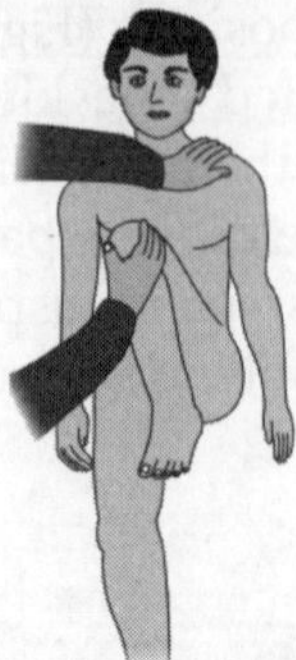

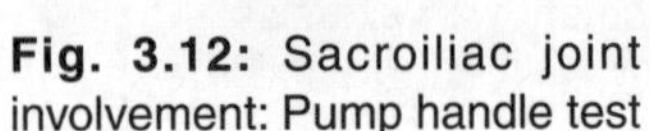

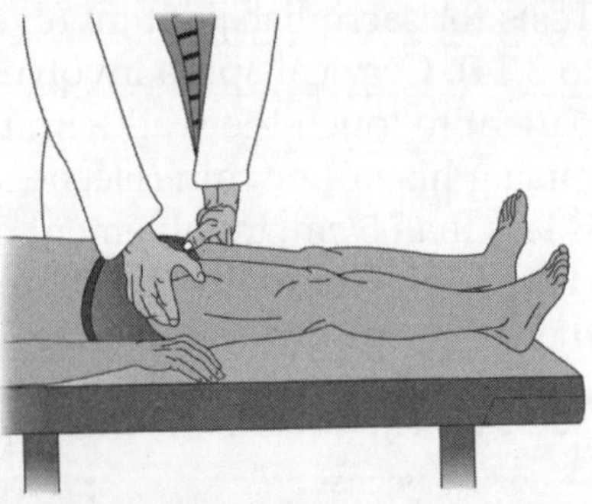

Fig. 3.12: Sacroiliac joint involvement: Pump handle test

Fig. 3.13: Sacroiliac joint involvement: Tested by the pelvic compression test

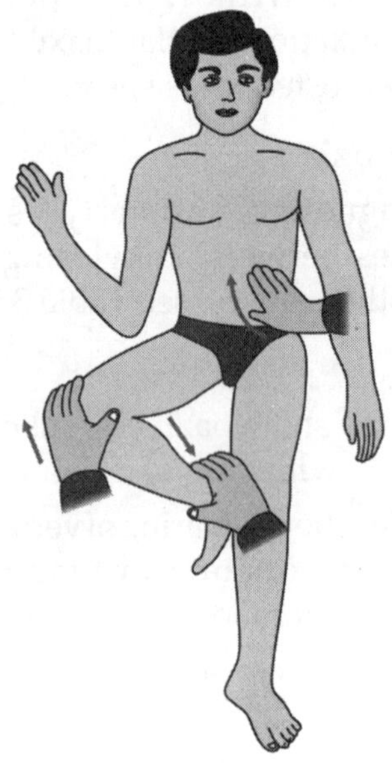

Fig. 3.14: Sacroiliac joint involvement: Fabre's test

- Patient education
- Family education
- Genetic counseling

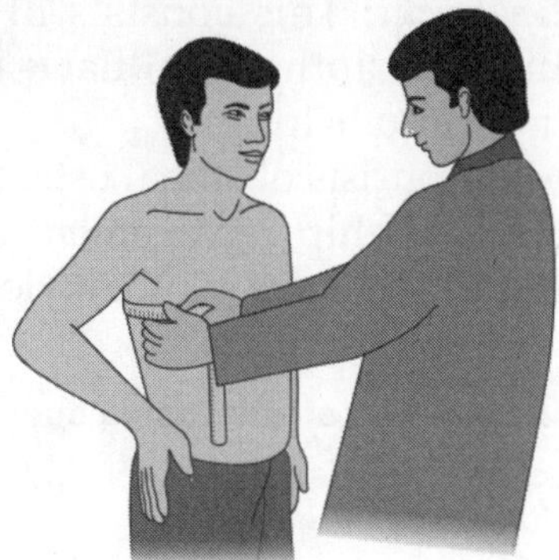

Fig. 3.15: Assessment of chest expansion in ankylosing spondylitis

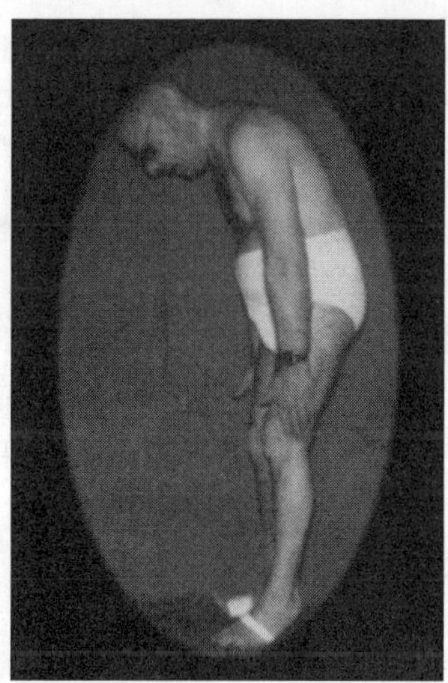

Fig. 3.16: This is how an ankylosing spondylitis patient looks (clinical photo)

- Avoid smoking
- Regular exercises, especially swimming is of tremendous help
- Physiotherapy and joint exercises
- Occupational therapy.

- *Conservative treatment:* This consists of rest, NSAIDs (indomethacin), physiotherapy, back exercises, etc. Radiotherapy may also help.
- *Surgical treatment:* Consists of spinal osteotomy to correct spine deformity, total hip replacement and total knee replacement for hip and knee joint ankylosis.

What is new in the treatment of ankylosing spondylitis?

Tumor necrosis factor antagonist etanercept (Enbrel) 25 mg twice weekly is being tried with successful results.

FIBROMYALGIA

Introduction

This is a condition where pain is characteristically described as "Charley horses" scattered all over the body. It falls in the gambit of muscular endurance disorders with a widespread musculoskeletal pain involving all the four quadrants of the body namely the right, left, above and below the waist (Fig. 3.18).

Incidence

After osteoarthritis, this is the most common rheumatological disorder. The overall incidence is 2–5 percent with women suffering 8–10 times more than man.

Causative Factors

- In 5–10 percent, it could be hereditary.
- In a majority, any condition that lowers the endurance of the muscles can trigger this condition. Notorious among them are sleep disorders (Loss of Stage IV delta wave sleep), trauma, connective tissue disorders, infections, etc.

Clinical Features

- *Pain:* Its features include widespread gnawing pains, with increased activity, stress or poor sleep.
- Fatigue, stiffness, arthralgia, headache, chest and abdominal pains, etc. are some of the other complaints.

Table 3.4: Differential diagnosis SSA

Disease	*Sex and age*	*Onset*	*Signs and symptoms*	*Joints involved*	*Extra-articular lesions*	*HLA-B_{27}*
Ankylosing spondylitis	Predominantly males < 40 years	Insidious	Low back pain, morning stiffness in heart, CNS disturbances, and pain > 3 months	Intervertebral joints	Uveitis, conduction defects pulmonary complications	94%
Psoriatic arthritis	Predominantly females > 50 years	Variable	Pain and stiffness on affected joints	Distal and proximal IP joints	Uveitis, conjunctivitis, urethritis, and skin lesions	100%
Reiter's disease	Predominantly females 16–35 years	Sudden	Pain and stiffness of affected joints, diarrhea, dysuria, etc.	Weight bearing joints (knee and ankle)	Conjunctivitis, uveitis, buccal erosions, urethritis	83%
Enteropathic arthropathies (Crohn's disease, ulcerative colitis, Whipple's disease)	Predominantly males Age group is not clear	Variable	Pain and stiffness of the affected joints, weight loss, diarrhea, abdominal pain	Knee, ankle (most common), shoulder wrist, elbow also involved	Aphthous ulcers, uveitis, erythema nodosum	50%
Behçet's Syndrome	Predominantly males 15–40 years	Variable	Pain and stiffness of affected joints	Knee, hand, ankle and wrist joints are primarily affected. There is involvement of elbow, shoulder and hip joints	Painful oral ulcers, genital ulcers, ocular lesions, Skin lesions.	16%

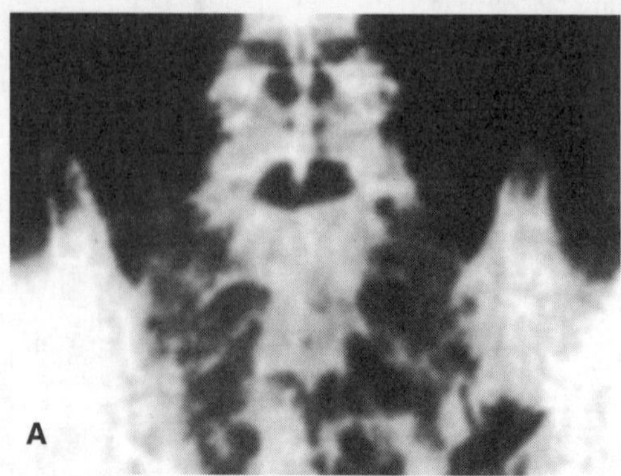

Fig. 3.17A: Radiograph showing sacroiliac joint sclerosis in ankylosing spondylitis

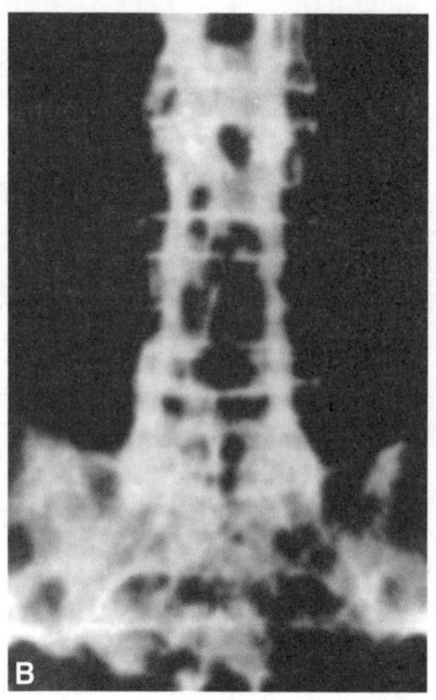

Fig. 3.17B: Radiograph showing bamboo spine in ankylosing spondylitis

Diagnostic Criteria

- Widespread pain for at least three months in all the four quadrants of the body
- Pain should be elicited in at least 11/18 established tender points when a digital pressure of 4 kg is applied (Fig. 3.19).

Table 3.5: Differential diagnosis of ankylosing spondylitis with other causes of backache

	Amkylosing Spondylitis	*Backache due to other causes*
Morning stiffness	Present	Nil or minimal
Effect of inactivity	Aggravates pain and stiffness	Relieves pain
Effect of physical activity	Relieves pain	Aggravates pain
Limitation of spine movements	In all directions	Only in some direction

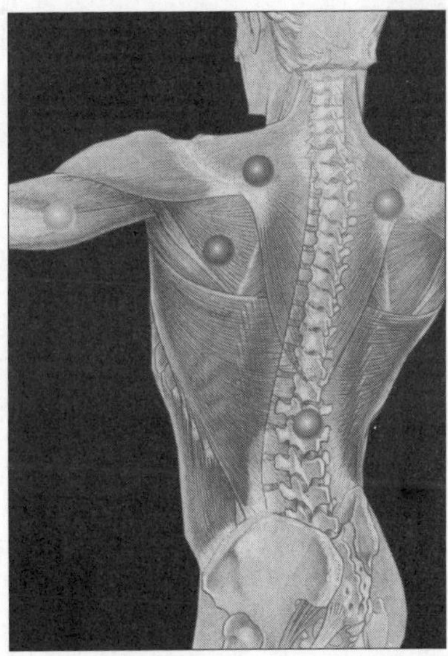

Fig. 3.18: Sites of tenderness in fibromyalgia

Treatment

A multidisciplinary approach seems to be an effective strategy in tackling this troublesome condition namely:

- *Initial phase*: Treat the underlying cause like sleep disorders, infection, connective tissue disorders, etc.
- *Second phase*: Myofascial release, massage and physical therapy are used to relieve the pain at the tender areas

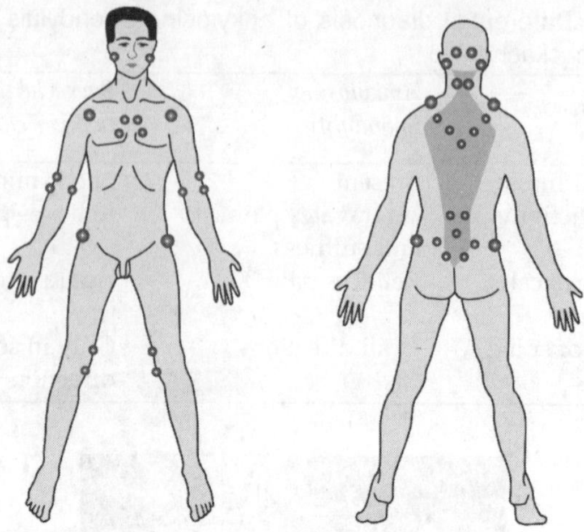

Fig. 3.19: Most common localization of tender points in fibromyalgia. Adapted from Mau (circles) and Moll (shadowed area)

- *Final phase:* Aerobic exercises are advocated to improve the muscle endurance.

Alternative Therapies

- *Diet therapy*: A diet rich in protein, amino acids and minerals are recommended.
- *Injection therapy*: A trigger point injection into the tender area with dry needling or injection, normal saline, local anesthetic and steroid injection helps.
- *Physiotherapy*: Ultrasound, SWD, TENS, manipulations and massage are useful adjunctive measures.
- *Acupressure*: Stimulating the reflex points and specific points helps to lower the pain.

CRYSTALLINE ARTHROPATHIES

This group includes two interesting clinical entities:

1. Monosodium urate arthropathies (gout) (Fig. 3.20).
2. Calcium pyrophosphate deposition disease (CPPD).

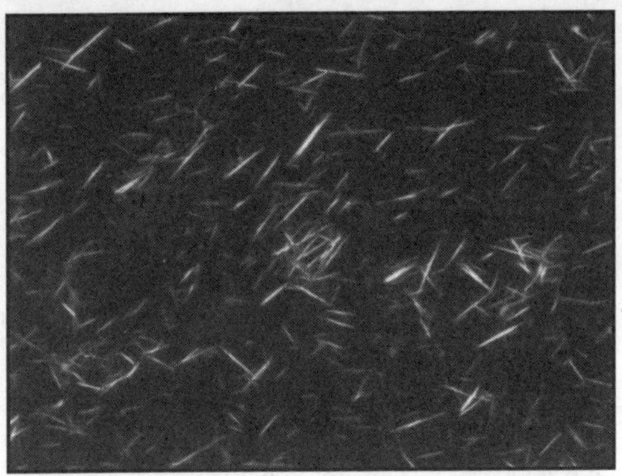

Fig. 3.20: Monosodium urate crystals viewed through a polarizing microscope

MONOSODIUM URATE ARTHROPATHY (GOUT)

This is known as *gout* and may manifest itself as *acute* or *chronic*.

Sites

It is usually monoarticular and the first metatarsophalangeal joint is the most common site of involvement (75%). Ankle, knee, wrist, fingers and elbow are other joints affected (Figs 3.21A and B). *Distal and lower extremity joints are involved more often.*

Role of Hyperuricemia

Gout is usually associated with hyperuricemia and may be associated with hypertension, obesity and atherosclerosis.

Did you know?

Gout is a disease of

- Affluence
- Alcoholism
- Obesity
- Old age
- Diuretic treatment

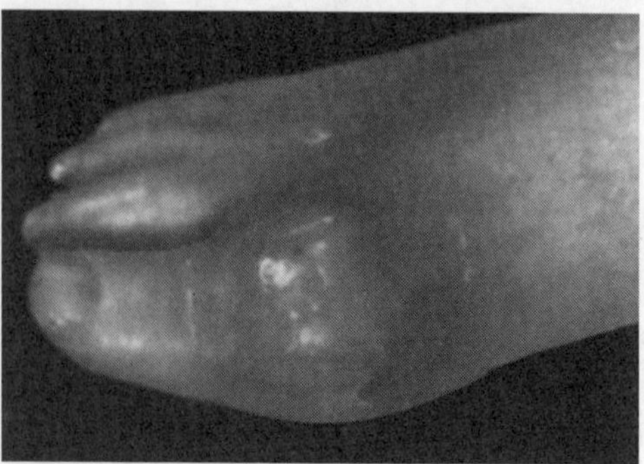

Fig. 3.21A: Features of acute gout (clinical photo)

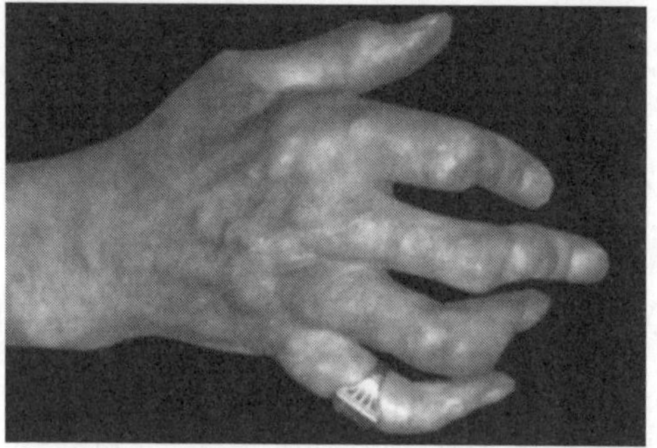

Fig. 3.21B: Features of chronic gout (clinical photo)

Incidence

It is about 0.3/1000 population.

Age

- Men — after mid-twenties.
- Women — after menopause.

Clinical Features

It has an abrupt onset. The patient may complain of pain, swelling, tenderness and increased temperature of the first metatarsophalangeal joint. Frequent gouty attacks disturb the sleep. Sometimes the inflammation is so gross that it may resemble cellulitis. Attacks are provoked by surgery, trauma, etc. Mild attacks resolve spontaneously within two days, more severe attacks may last for 7–10 days.

Gout has two extremes. At one end is obese alcoholic with family history of gout and no tophi while at the other extreme is an old, frail, taking thiazide diuretics and with tophi.

TOPHI These are deposits of monosodium urate crystals over pinnae, elbows Achilles tendon, distal IP joints is elderly patients.

Investigations

Laboratory investigations show leucocytosis and ESR is increased. Synovial fluid study is done under polarized microscopy for the presence of monosodium urate crystals. *This is the most important diagnostic method* (Fig. 3.20). Raised SUA level may be found.

Radiology

It is usually normal but may provide a helpful clue to detect chondrocalcinosis.

Treatment

Conservative method is the mainstay of treatment. The following measures are recommended: Indomethacin 75–100 mg oral initially. Later, it is given as 50 mg every 6 hours. As the attack subsides, the drug may be tapered off. Intra-articular steroid also helps. Recurrent gouty arthritic attacks can be prevented by prophylaxis with colchicines (0.5 mg BD) or indomethacin (25–50 mg everyday). When the above two drugs do not help, Allopurinol is indicated on a long-term basis.

Remember the Diagnostic Features of Gout

*Attacks (**4Rs**)*

- **R**apid onset
- **R**ecurrent
- **R**arely seen > 10 days
- Remissions

*Joints (remember the mnemonic **FRAME**)*

- **F**irst MTP joint involved

- **R**ed hot joint
- **A**rticular involvement usually single
- **M**any urate crystals within neutrophils is joint fluid
- **E**xtreme pain.

Non-articular features

- Hyperuricemia
- Tophi (in elderly).

The drugs used in the prevention and treatment of gout:

- Indomethacin
- Colchicines prevention
- Allopurinol
- Steroids.

Aspiration of the affected joint and intra-articular steroid injection terminates as acute attack of gout.

PSEUDOGOUT (CPPD)

Pseudogout is due to deposition of calcium pyrophosphate in the joints. Larger joints are more affected and 50 percent involve the knee joints unlike in gout (Fig. 3.22). Other areas commonly involved are elbows, wrists, ankles, shoulder and hip. Synovial fluid study under polarized microscopy reveals CPP crystals. The disease is not as severe as gout and is much rarer.

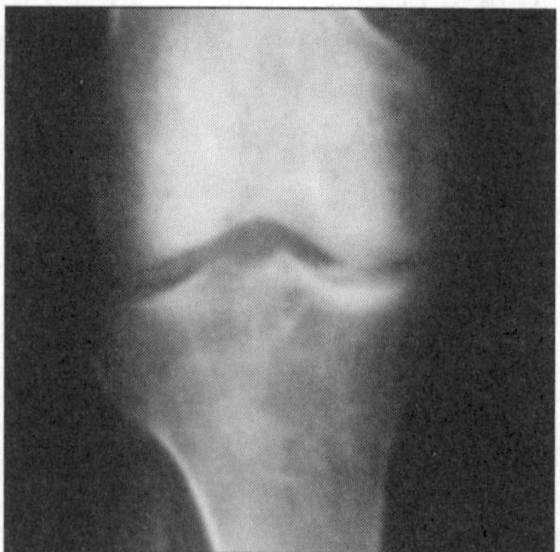

Fig. 3.22: Radiograph showing pseudogout in knee joint

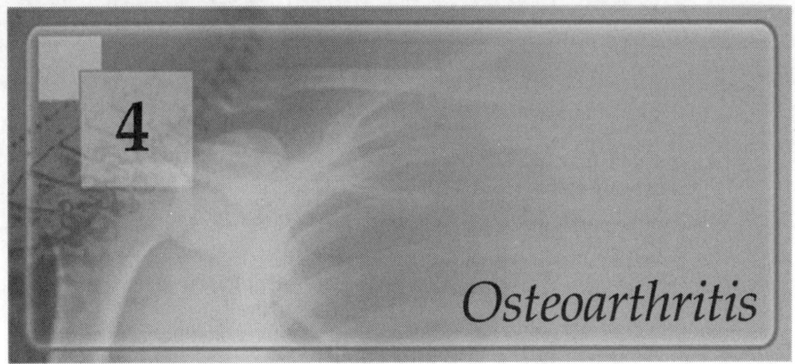

This chapter deals with important degenerative problems in orthopedics

OSTEOARTHRITIS OF THE KNEE

Definition

It is defined as a degenerative, non-inflammatory joint disease characterized by destruction of articular cartilage and formation of new bone at the joint surfaces and margins.

The term osteoarthritis was coined by *John Spendon*. However, it is a misnomer and the right term is osteoarthrosis or degenerative joint disease. It could be primary or secondary and the former is more common.

Osteoarthritis affects the synovial joints, though it can affect any joint, it is more common in the weight bearing joints like the hip, knee, spine, etc. (Fig. 4.1).

PRIMARY OSTEOARTHRITIS OF THE KNEE

(Also called idiopathic)

Etiological causes for primary osteoarthritis: Though exact cause is not known, the following factors are suspected to play an important role in the causation of primary osteoarthritis—obesity, genetics and heredity, occupation involving prolonged standing, sports, multiple endocrinal disorders and multiple metabolic disorders.

Note: Genetic tendency in OA knee is twice as strong as OA hip.

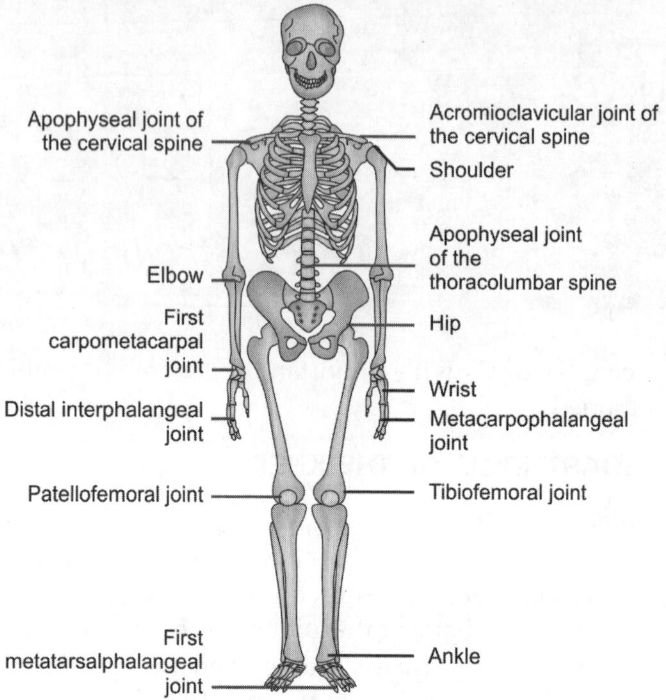

Fig. 4.1: Sites of primary osteoarthritis

Risk Factors: There are many risk factors that predispose to the development of this condition. The important ones are listed in the box on the next page.

Features

- It commonly affects the knee joint.
- All races are susceptible.
- Common in older age groups.
- Eighty percent of people are affected by 40 years, but only 40 percent show symptoms.
- It causes varus deformity of the knee in the late stages (Fig. 4.2).
- More than 50 percent have bilateral OA knee.

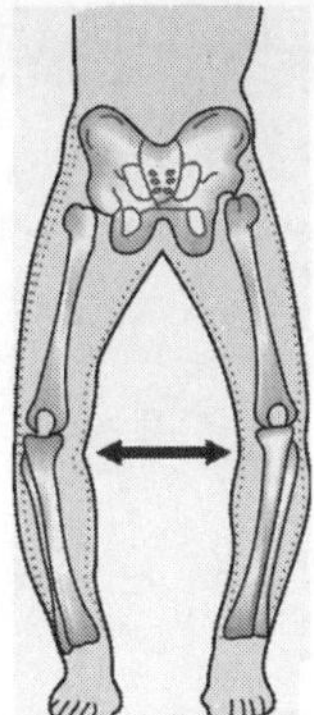

Fig. 4.2: Genu varum deformity in advanced osteoarthritis of knee

Quick facts: Osteoarthritis

Who is prone to get osteoarthritis?

- Middle-aged patients
- Women have a greater tendency than men do
- One in three people over 60 years are affected and more than three in four persons over the age of seventy show some radiographic evidence of the condition
- Very rarely it can be seen in younger people.

What are the typical symptoms of osteoarthritis?

- Pain
- Early morning stiffness
- Restricted range of joint movements
- Swelling of the joints.

What joints are usually affected?

- Weight bearing joints like hip, knee, ankle, etc.
- Spine
- Fingers.

What causes osteoarthritis?

- Age more than 40 years
- Female
- Hereditary conditions
- Previous joint injuries
- Obesity
- Diseases of the joints
- Poor posture
- Occupational stress
- A combination of the above factors.

Note: The only factor, which can be modified, is obesity.

How to make a diagnosis?

- Physical examination
- Symptomatology
- Radiography
- Blood tests
- CT scan and MRI.

Remember the risk factors

O – Obesity
S – Senility or old age
T – Trauma
E – Emotional stress
O – Osteoporosis
A – Alcohol
R – Rigorous lifestyles
T – Taxing professions
H – Hormonal imbalances
R – Repetitive injuries
I – Indian cultural habits
T – Axing sports
I – Improper postural habits
S – Smoking

Sequence of pathological events in osteoarthritis: The disease process usually begins in the anteromedial compartment of the knee joint.

Fibrillation due to loss of water of the weight bearing articular cartilage is seen in early stages of the disease followed by complete loss of articular cartilage. This puts enormous pressure on the underlying bone, which causes sclerosis and later eburnation. Cysts may develop in the subchondral area due to microfractures that degenerate. New bone formation takes place and results in osteophyte formation (Figs 4.3A to C).

Note: OA is characterized by architectural deterioration of articular cartilage and formation of new bone at the joint surfaces.

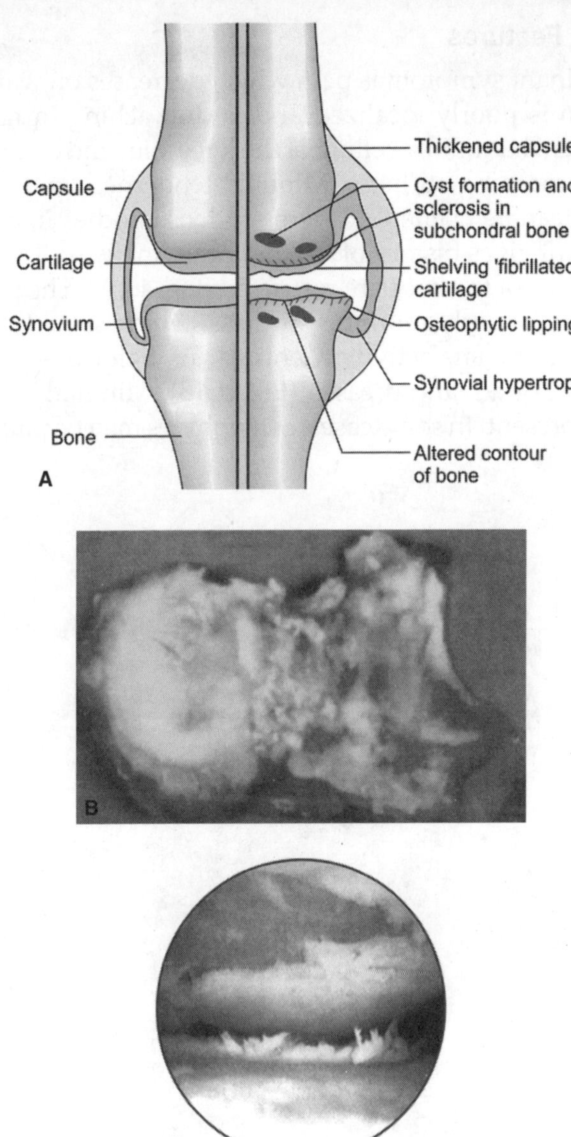

Figs 4.3A to C: (A) Pathological features of osteoarthritis knee, (B) Pathological specimen showing destruction of articular cartilage in OA knee, (C) Arthroscopic view of degenerated cartilage in OA knee

Clinical Features

Predominant symptom is pain which decreases on walking. The pain is poorly localized and is dull aching in nature. The patient has mild swelling of the knee joint and complains of early morning stiffness. Minimal tenderness and coarse crepitus can be elicited. If there are loose bodies in a joint, the patient gives history of locking or giving way. Terminal movements of the knee are restricted (Fig. 4.4A). The patient complains of early morning stiffness, which subsides over the day after some activity. Genu varum deformity may be seen in very advanced cases (Fig. 4.4B). Minimal effusion may be present. In some cases, osteophytes may be palpable.

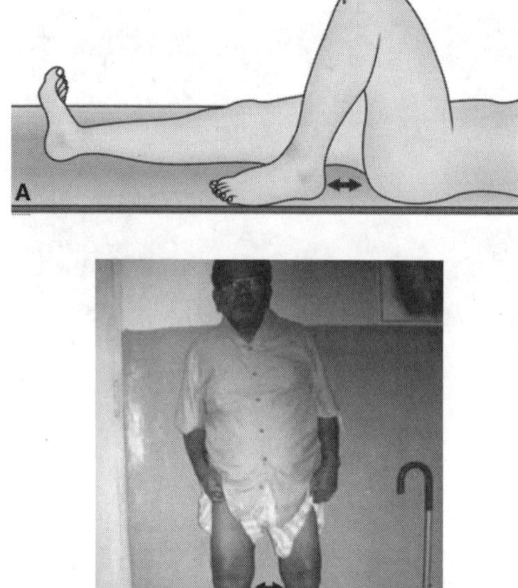

Figs 4.4A and B: (A) Loss of terminal flexion in osteoarthritis knee, (B) Genu varum deformity (clinical photo)

Do you know the sources of pain in OA knee?

Well, it could be from

- Inflamed synovium
- Microfracture of subchondral bone
- Periosteum stretching by osteophytes
- Venous congestion in intraosseous compartment
- Joint distension
- Muscle spasm
- Bursal inflammations
- Affered joint mechanics
- Mental depression.

Quick facts: About complaints in OA knee

- Pain limits walking distance and capacity to work
- Limp
- Difficulty to knee, get up from the chairs, getting in and out of the car
- Descend and ascend the stairs
- Limits capacity to work, even housework.

Examination of the patient in OA knee

Standing

→ From front
→ Deformity (Knock knee—Uncommon Bowleg—Common)
→ Early stages → Correctible by manual stress (Indicates unilateral OA)
→ Late stages → Not correctible (Bilateral) TKR needed

→ From the sides
→ Knee will not straighten fully (due to fibrous and capsular contractures)

Criteria and Classification of OA Knee (American College of Rheumatology—ACR)

(For medical readers only)

Clinical

1. Knee pain for most days of prior month.
2. Crepitus on active joint motion.
3. Morning stiffness equal and not more than 30 minutes in duration.
4. Age equal to more than 38 years.
5. Bony enlargement of the knee on examination.

Clinical and Radiological

1. Knee pain for most days of the prior month.
2. Osteophytes at joint margins.
3. Synovial fluid typical of OA knee.
4. Age—40 years.
5. Morning stiffness equal and not more than 30 minutes.
6. Crepitus on active joint motion.

OA is present (Clinical)

1, 2, 3, 4 or 1, 2, 5 or 1, 4, 5

OA Present (clinical and radiological)

1, 2 or 1, 3, 5, 6 or 1, 4, 5, 6. Modified from Attman (1986) and Atman (1991).

Investigations

Laboratory investigations are usually within normal limits.

Radiological examination of the knee joint is the most important diagnostic tool. The following are the radiological features seen in osteoarthritis (Figs 4.5A and B) of the knee.

- Loss of joint space (due to destruction of articular cartilage).
- Sclerosis (due to increase cellularity and bone deposition).

- Subchondral cysts (due to synovial fluid intrusion into the bone).
- Osteophytes (due to revascularization of remaining cartilage and capsular traction).
- Bony collapse (due to compression of weakened bone).
- Loose bodies (due to fragmentation of osteochondral surface).
- Deformity and malalignment (due to destruction of capsules and ligaments).

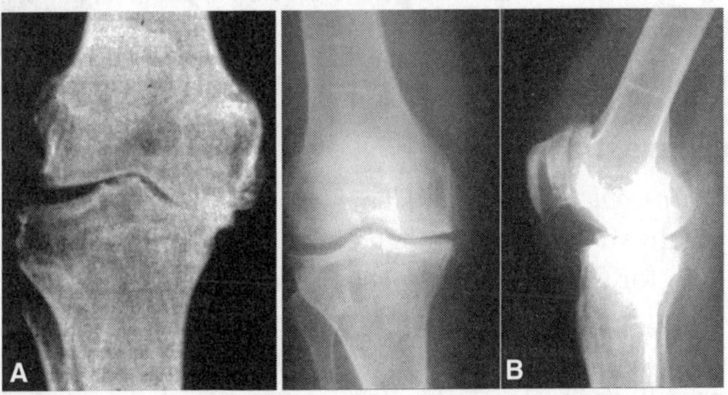

Figs 4.5A and B: (A) Radiograph showing knee joint showing loss of joint space, osteophytes, subchondral sclerosis and varus deformity, (B) Radiograph showing Tri-compartmental OA knee

Kellegren and Lawrence Radiological Grading

Grade I: Doubtful narrowing of joint space and possible osteophyte lipping.

Grade II: Definite osteophytes and possible narrowing of the joint space.

Grade III: Moderate multiple osteophytes, definite narrowing of joint space and some sclerosis and possible deformity of the bone ends.

Grade IV: Large osteophytes, marked narrowing of joint space, severe sclerosis and definite deformity of the bone ends.

Pitfalls of X-rays in OA Knee

- Not reliable in about 15 percent of the cases.
- Weight bearing AP and lateral views are desired.
- Only 40 percent of the people with severe X-ray changes experience pain.

Radiological Classification of OA Knee (Ahlbach) AP weight Bearing and Lateral Views

Type I : Joint space narrowing.
Type II : Total loss of joint space.
Type III : < 5 mm tibial erosion but posterior part of the plateau intact.
Type IV : > 5 mm tibial erosion and erosion of posterior plateau.
Type V : Subluxation.

Note: Grades IV and V: TKR is the line of treatment.

Other Investigations

- *Arthroscopic examination:* This allows direct inspection and visualization of the damaged joint surfaces. But arthroscopy alone for diagnostic purposes is rarely used (Fig. 4.3C).
- Synovial fluid analysis shows non-inflammatory picture. Bone scan shows increased uptake of technetium-99m, MRI and CT scan also helps to diagnose, subchondral cysts, osteophytes, etc. (Fig. 4.6).

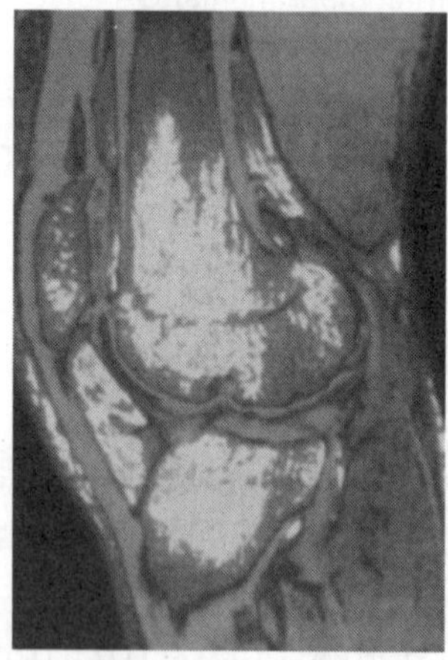

Fig. 4.6: MRI OA knee

Treatment

- Before beginning the treatment, the diagnosis of OA is a must. ACR diagnostic criteria for OA knee to be followed.
- Treatment to be individualized and tailored to severity.
- Multiple strategies may be required in most of the cases.

ACR Guidelines: Traditional Format

- Knee pain.
- Radiographic osteophytes.
- At least one of the following three:
  - Age greater than 50 years.
  - Morning stiffness less than or equal to 30 minutes.
  - Crepitus on motion.

Aims of Treatment of OA Knee

It can be best illustrated by 4 Rs:

- **R**elieve pain.
- **R**estore function.
- **R**educe disability if any
- **R**ehabilitation.

Conservative Methods

This forms the mainstay of management in osteoarthritis of the knee. About 50 percent of patients respond to conservative treatment, which consists of the following measures.

Nonpharmacological Treatment

This is the initial and main stay of treatment in OA knees. The important recommendations of ACR are:

- Self education—Educating the patient and his relatives measures about the disease is the most important aspect of the nonpharmacological treatment and should be done first.
- Health professional social support
- Weight loss

- Physiotherapy
- Therapuetic exercises
- Assistive devices
- Occupational therapy
- Aerobic exercise program
- Strengthening of the quadriceps
- Supervised fitness walking program
- Swimming/hydrotherapy
- Modifications of activity of daily living.

Mechanical aids

- Cane in the contralateral hand
- Mechanical aids
- Medial taping of the patella in PF diseases
- Light weight knee braces in TF diseases. Now let us analyse the treatment methods:

Components of Therapeutic Exercise

- *Range of motion and flexibility:* Soft tissue flexibility of both contractile (muscle, tendon) and noncontractile tissues (capsule, ligaments) is affected by arthritis and inactivity. Joint stiffness and soft tissue shortening can be reduced with appropriate range of motion (ROM) and stretching exercises.
- *Muscle strengthening:* All aspects of muscle strength (strength, endurance, power) can be impacted as a result of intra-articular and extra-articular inflammatory processes, disuse, reflex inhibition in response to pain and joint effusion, decreased protective muscular reflexes, loss of mechanical integrity around the joint, and even medication side effects. Muscle strengthening exercises helps to overcome these problems.
- *Quadriceps exercises:* Strengthening of quadriceps musculature with either isometric or isotonic, resistive exercises was associated with significant improvement in quadriceps strength, knee pain, and function.

- *Aerobic (cardiovascular) exercise:* Persons with arthritis tend to be less fit than noninvolved peers. However, there is strong evidence for the role of regular and vigorous exercise to improve all components of physical fitness, including cardiovascular fitness and endurance even in people with arthritis. Most studies have limited their interventions to walking, stationary bicycling, aerobic dancing, aquatic exercise, and circuit training at moderate intensity levels.
- *Body awareness exercise:* Body awareness exercises address posture, core stability, balance, proprioception, coordination, and relaxation. Benefits of these exercises include decreased risks for falls and musculoskeletal injury.
- *Recreational and community:* Based exercise the advantages of community-based exercise include a focus on wellness, increased socialization, and peer support. As well, the greater variety in exercise facilities, classes, and equipment may enhance motivation and ongoing adherence. Aquatic exercises are a good choice for individuals with arthritis, particularly those with lower extremity involvement.

Physiotherapy

Physical modalities that may contribute to pain relief include the application of superficial heat (hot packs, heating pads, hot water bottles, or paraffin) and/or cold (cold packs or ice packs).

Weight Loss

Obesity is a risk factor for the development of OA, and is associated with radiological progression of the disease, and disability. When people walk, 3–6 times their body weight is transferred across the knee joint; any excess weight should be multiplied by this factor to estimate the excess force across the knee joint of overweight people.

In managing OA, weight reduction should be a key goal. Exercise plays a role, but pain and disability can make it difficult for patients to exercise sufficiently to lose weight. Weight loss can be achieved with regular sessions with a dietitian who can provide instruction on reducing caloric intake and the use of food diaries, and cognitive-behavioral modification to change dietary habits.

Pharmacologic Drugs

- *Nonopioid analgesics, e.g. acetaminophen:* This is the drug of first choice. Up to 4 gm/day can be given.
- *NSAIDs:* If patients fail to respond to paracetamol or other oral or topical analgesics, then the use of an NSAID is indicated.
- *Opioid analgesics:* These can be tried if patients fail to respond to paracetamol and NSAIDs
- *Food supplementation:* Glucosamine and Chondroitin sulfate: Can reduce 20–25 percent pain in mild to moderate OA. Over the counter food supplements, 1500 mg/day for at least 3 months.
- *Intra-articular steroids:* This is indicated if there is effusion and there are signs of inflammation
- *Viscosupplementation:* Injection of hyaluronic acid into the joint. Once a week for 3 weeks. Adverse reactions in 2–3 percent.
- *Topical analgesics:* These are indicated in the following situations:
  - If patients do not respond to oral analgesics.
  - If patients do not wish to take systemic drugs.
  - Can be used as a monotherapy or adjunct.
  - Capsaicin cream – 4 times a day.

Viscosuplementation in OA knee?

Viscosuplementation (Intra-articular hyaluronan therapy): This procedure consists of removal of pathologic osteoarthritis synovial fluid and replacement of hyaluronan-based products that restore the molecular weight and concentration of hyaluronan to normal values that is reduced in OA knee.

Hyaluronan helps in joint lubrication, buffers load transmission, imparts anti-inflammatory properties to synovial fluid.

Indications for Intra-articular Hyaluronic Acid Injection

- Failed conservative treatment
- If there are major risk factors for surgery
- Failed intra-articular steroid injections
- Advanced osteoarthritis.

By combining steroid injection with joint lavage, OA patients get more effective pain relief than with either therapy alone and pain could reduce for as long as 24 weeks.

Mechanical Aids

They reduce the load on the knee joint and provides support to the weak knees. The following are used in OA knees:

- Cane
- Shoe inserts
- *Shoe supplements:* Good shock absorber, good mediolateral support, adequate arch support, calcaneal cushion.
- *Lateral heel wedges:* To reduce pain of medial tibiofemoral joint OA.
- Knee brace and support in varus knees.

Alternative Therapies

- Acupuncture
- Bio-feedback
- Naturopathy
- Aquatic physical therapy
- Massage
- Acupressure
- Tai Chi
- Balenotherapy
- Yoga

The proponents of alternative therapies claim good results from their respective interventions. The results are good in the hands of experts.

Surgery

Indications for Surgery

- Pain refractory to conservative measures.
- History of frequent locking episodes.
- Hemarthrosis due to loose bodies or osteochondral fractures.
- Deformity, usually genu varum.
- Joint instability.
- Progressive limitation of knee motion.

Surgical Methods

- *Excision of osteophytes* is rarely done alone.
- *Excision of loose bodies, meniscectomy, synovectomy,* and *reconstruction or joint debridement* are best done by arthroscopy.
- *Proximal tibial osteotomy (Slocum's):* Indicated for unicompartmental osteoarthritis of knee with pain and also to correct varus (less than 15°) or valgus deformity (less than 12°). Pain is decreased in 80 percent of the cases following surgery as osteotomy changes the line of weightbearing and brings the more normal surface to carry out the function of load transmission (Fig. 4.7). Mean failure rate is 40 percent at 4 years.
- *Distal femoral osteotomy* is indicated when varus or valgus deformity of the knee is more than 12–15°.
- *Chondral resurfacing procedure*
  - *Autologous chondrocyte grafting*: Autologous chondrocytes from the patient's knee are cultured for two weeks, reinserted under a patch of periosteum.
  - *Mosaic plasty*: Spare autologous hyaline cartilage from other areas of knee is inserted into the defect.
- *Arthroscopic debridement:* This is a successful palliative, temporizing treatment of OA knee.
- *Total knee arthroplasty:* This is indicated when both the compartments of the knee joint are destroyed or if valgus

or varus deformity is more than 15°. It is also indicated in failed conservative treatment (Figs 4.8 and 4.9).

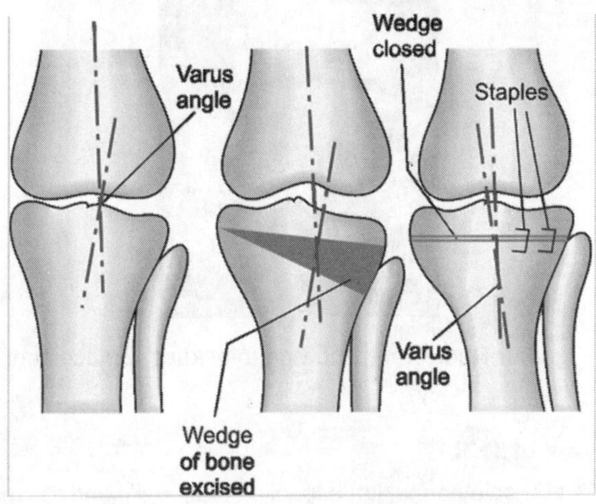

Fig. 4.7: Valgus high tibial osteotomy

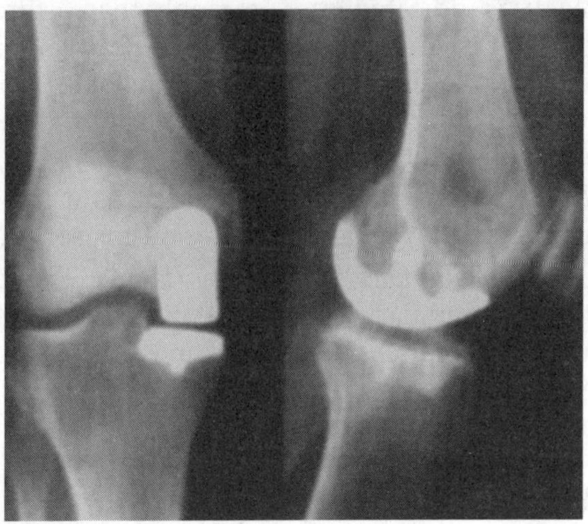

Fig. 4.8: Radiographs showing unicondylar knee replacement

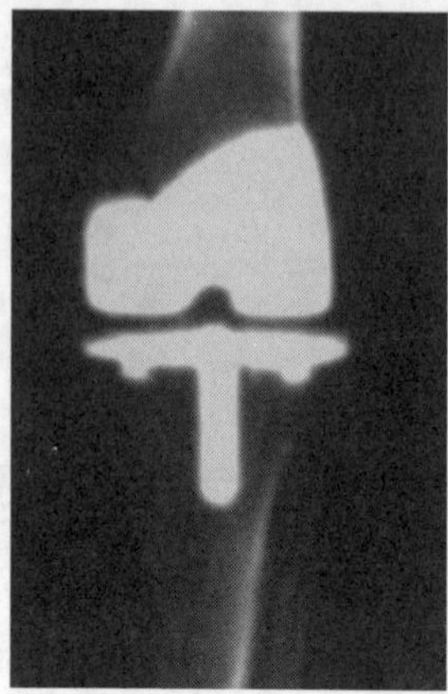

Fig. 4.9: Radiograph showing total knee replacement

Limitations of TKR

- Only 1 in 6-gain normal knee function after TKR, and the rest have residual symptoms.
- Full flexion not regained.
- Anterior wound prevents kneeling.

- *Arthrodesis* is indicated less commonly than arthroplasty. If the patient is young and involved in heavy occupation, arthrodesis is indicated to give him a stable and strong knee. However, arthrodesis results in a stiff knee, which is a severe disability.
- *Patellectomy:* It is rarely done except as a last resort. Contemplated in osteoarthritis present for several years.
- *Unicompartmental knee arthroplasty (UKA):* This is again regaining its popularity over tibial osteotomy in treating unicompartmental OA, as it helps in early postoperative rehabilitation.

Macquet's HTO (High tibial osteotomy) this is another useful procedure

Did you know?

Steindler described osteotomy for OA knee in 1940.

SECONDARY OSTEOARTHRITIS OF THE KNEE

It is generally observed that secondary osteoarthritis occurs in the younger age groups and is more severe than the primary. Apart from all the features of osteoarthritis, secondary osteoarthritis has the features of the corresponding etiological condition.

The causes for secondary osteoarthritis of the knee are as follows:

- Obesity.
- Valgus and varus deformities of the knee.
- Intra-articular fractures of the knee, etc.
- Rheumatoid arthritis, infection, trauma, TB, etc.
- Hyperparathyroidism.
- Hemophilia.
- Syringomyelia.
- Neurological disease like diabetes.
- Overuse of intra-articular steroid therapy.

Remember

Major complications of osteoarthritis of knee

- Joint deformities
- Subluxation
- Ankylosis
- Intra-articular loose bodies.

Os in osteoarthritis of the knee

- **O**besity
- **O**ccupation
- **O**ver 40 years of age
- **O**ther predisposing joint diseases
- **O**steophytes main characteristic feature of osteoarthritis
- **O**utward deviation of knee
- **O**steotomy required correcting bone deformities.

OSTEOARTHRITIS OF THE HIP

(Familiarly Called as Malum Coxa Senilis)

This is second in frequency to knee joint, and it could be primary or secondary.

PRIMARY OSTEOARTHRITIS OF THE HIP

This is idiopathic and forms 50 percent of the osteoarthritis of the hip. In this variety, the exact cause is not known and the causative factors suspected are increased anteversion, and trabecular microfracture causing stiffening of the subchondral bone.

SECONDARY OSTEOARTHRITIS OF THE HIP

The following factors are responsible for the development of secondary osteoarthritis of the hip joint.

- *Incongruity of the articular surface,* e.g. trauma, Perthe's, CDH, slipped epiphysis.
- *Instability of the hip,* e.g. subluxation.
- *Concentration of pressure load,* e.g. coxa vara, anteversion.
- *Direct injury,* e.g. infection, trauma.
- *Constitutional causes,* e.g. obesity, hyperthyroidism.
- Bone diseases like AVN, rheumatoid arthritis, etc.

Remember

About secondary osteoarthritis

- Progress is relentless.
- Occurs in younger age group.
- Nonsurgical treatment is futile.
- If surgery is prolonged for long, the optimal time for surgery is missed.

Pathology

The changes in the articular cartilage vary from fibrillation to complete destruction depending on the severity of osteoarthritis. The synovium is thick and congested. The subchondral bone shows sclerosis and cyst formation. The capsule is thick and fibrosed. New bone growth results in osteophyte formation in areas not under pressure.

Clinical Features

In osteoarthritis of the hip joint, the patient is asymptomatic in the early stages, later patient may complain of slight pain in the hip lasting for 1–2 days. Stiffness of the hip, muscle spasm, limp, restriction of terminal hip movements is the other complaints. As the disease advances, pain decreases, but the hip becomes more and more stiff. A mild flexion, adduction and external rotation deformity may be seen.

Radiographs

Primary Osteoarthritis

In the early stages, no changes are seen. In the later stages joint space is reduced, subchondral sclerosis, cysts, osteophytes, etc. may be seen (Figs 4.10A and B).

Secondary osteoarthritis: Apart from features of osteoarthritis, features of the predisposing causes are also seen.

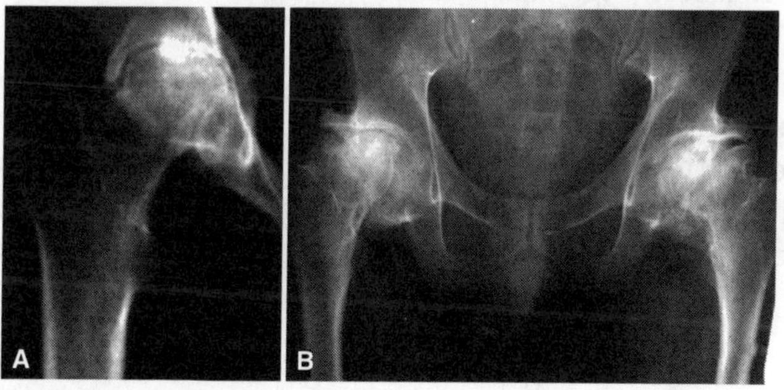

Figs 4.10A and B: (A) Radiograph showing osteoarthritis of hip, (B) Bilateral OA hip

Treatment Methods

Conservative Measures

Consist of rest, heat, NSAIDs, muscle relaxant, massage, traction, manipulation, intra-articular steroids, etc.

Surgical

Careful selection of the cases is done. Primary aim of surgery is relief of pain, while secondary aim is to restore movements, increase stability and deformity correction.

In the early stages of the disease when a fair amount of hip movements is still present, osteotomy helps while in the later stages it is total hip or resurfacing arthroplasties.

Osteotomy Methods

Pauwell's varus osteotomy: It is done if osteoarthritis is due to coxa valga.

Valgus osteotomy: This is more common and is done in adduction deformity of the hip.

Displacement osteotomy (Mc Murray's): This is indicated in severe osteoarthritis of hip with large osteophytes.

Osteotomy helps by changing the line of weight bearing and bringing the normal surface into the line of weight transmission (Figs 4.11A and B).

Hip Arthroplasties

In the late stages of osteoarthritis, in elderly and in restriction of flexion less than 70°, osteotomy is of no value. The choice is then between cup arthroplasty, arthrodesis, hemi-replacement arthroplasty and total hip replacement (Figs 4.12 and 4.13).

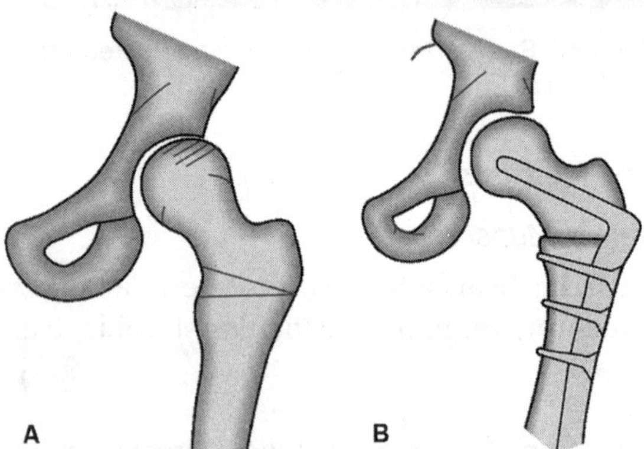

Figs 4.11A and B: Osteotomy for hip in osteoarthritis: (A) Before operation, (B) After operation

Resurfacement Arthroplasty

Birmingham hip resurfacing arthroplasty is emerging as an effective alternative to the conventional THR. Here only the diseased head is resurfaced and not resected. It preserves unaffected portion of the head and neck. It is indicated in slightly younger patient.

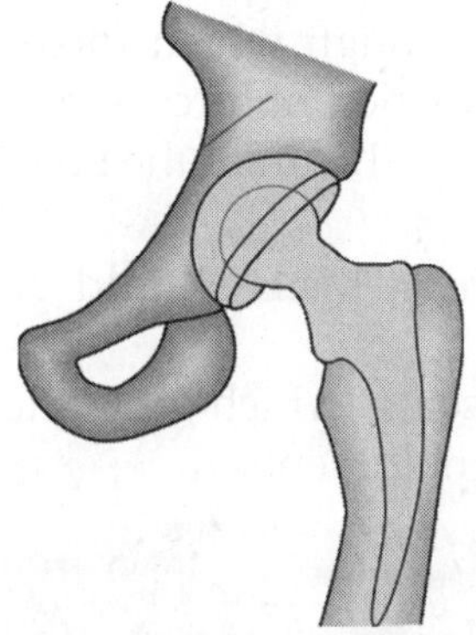

Fig. 4.12: Total hip replacement for osteoarthritis of hip

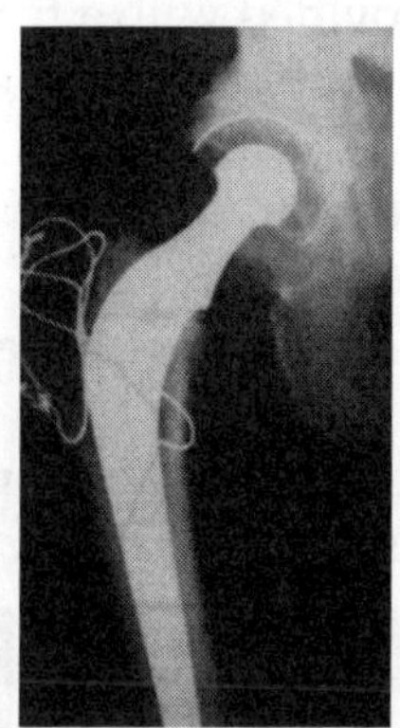

Fig. 4.13: Radiograph showing THR

Modifications of Activity of Daily Living in the Management of Osteoarthritis of Hip and Knee Joints

Simple changes around the home and daily activities causes dramatic improvement in the symptomatology of ostcoarthritis. The following are some of the measures:

- Use of higher chair, which require less effort to get in and get out, should be considered (Fig. 4.14A).
- Changes to be made in the bathroom:
  - Use of Western toilets and avoiding the Indian types.
  - To fit the bath aids to facilitate easy getting in getting out of a bath.
  - To fit railings next to the toilet and bath to facilitate ease of movement.
- Patients are advised to *climb* the stairs leading the *good leg* taking one stair at a time and to *descend* the stairs leading

with the *bad leg*, again taking one stair at a time (Fig. 4.14B).

- To reduce the force acting across the injured joint, the patient is advised to use a walking stick, which acts as a *third limb*. The stick should be held in the hand opposite to the affected hip or knee. Initially, it should be used around the home. The top of the stick should come up to the wrist when the patient stands and the tip should be provided with a firm rubber to avoid slipping. A walking stick, by providing a third limb through which forces can be transmitted, enables the reduction of force across the injured joint from peak values of 5–1.5 times the body weight (Fig. 4.14C).
- Footwear with hard soles and high heels should be avoided.
- Cars with raised platforms and seats, which facilitate easy getting in and getting out, should be used.

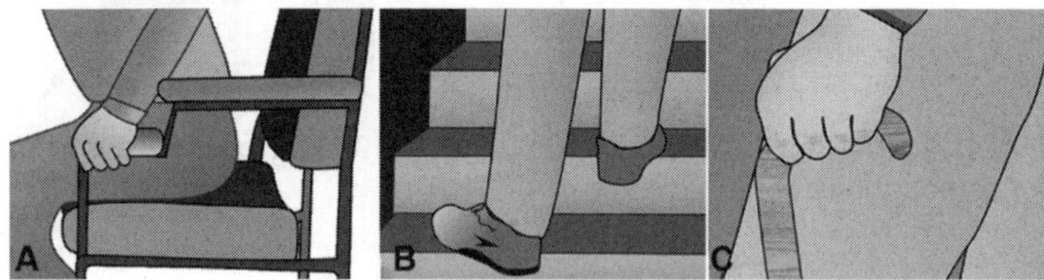

Figs 4.14A to C: Modification of living habits in the management of osteoarthritis of hip and knee: (A) Higher chairs, less effort, (B) Stairs often present a problem, and (C) Walking sticks of the right height

- If the patients are overweight, reduction in the weight helps to reduce the load on the joints.
- General advice when standing:
  - Keep as upright as possible as this helps to put equal weight on both the legs.
  - Avoid sitting on a low or soft chair.
  - Avoid curling up in bed.
  - To stretch the front of the thigh and hip, lie on the stomach at least once a day for 5–30 minutes.

- To use a walking stick when walking inside or outside the house (cane reduces load by 40–50%).
- To avoid uneven and rough ground or surfaces while walking.
- To wear comfortable footwears.

Role of Exercises in the Management of Osteoarthritis of the Hip and Knee

Exercises from the mainstay of the patients own contribution in the treatment of osteoarthritis of the hip and knee.

Quick facts

Aims of the exercises in osteoarthritis hip and knee

- To increase the range of movements.
- To increase stability and shock absorption.
- To prevent deformity.
- To improve posture.
- To reduce pain and stiffness.

Rules of the exercises

- Build-up the exercises gradually.
- Avoid rough ground while exercising.
- To take warm baths before starting the exercises.
- To perform the exercises 20 times each twice a day and later four times a day.

Types of Exercises in Osteoarthritis of Hip

Exercises Lying on the Back (Figs 4.15A to D)

- *Pelvic tilt:* Tighten the thigh and buttock muscles, pushing the knees flat, hold for a count of five and relax (Fig. 4.15A).
- *Pelvic lift:* Bend both the knees up, push on the feet and lift, hold for a count of five and relax (Fig. 4.15B).
- *Leg stretch:* Push one leg along the floor as though you are trying to make it longer than the other. Hold for a count of five and then repeat with the other leg (Fig. 4.15C).
- *Alternate leg rising:* Keeping the knees straight, lift alternate legs six inches from the ground (Fig. 4.15D).

Exercises Lying on your Side, with the Painful Hip up (Figs 4.16A to C)

- *Side leg rising:* Keep the top leg straight and lift it up as high as possible, hold for a count of five and relax (Figs 4.16B and C).
- *Knee and hip flexion:* Bend the hip and knee of the top leg forwards, and hold for a count of five. Then straighten the leg and stretch backwards as far as it will go, hold for a count of five, then relax (Fig. 4.16A).

Exercises in Sitting Posture (Figs 4.17A and B)

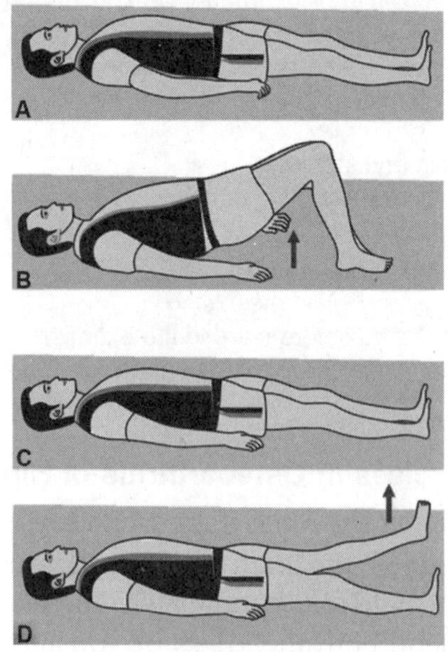

Figs 4.15A to D: Exercises on lying back: (A) Pelvic tilt, (B) Pelvic lift, (C) Leg stretch, and (D) Alternate leg raising

- *Knees together, feet apart:* Keep the knees together and move the feet apart, hold for a count of five then relax (Fig. 4.17A).

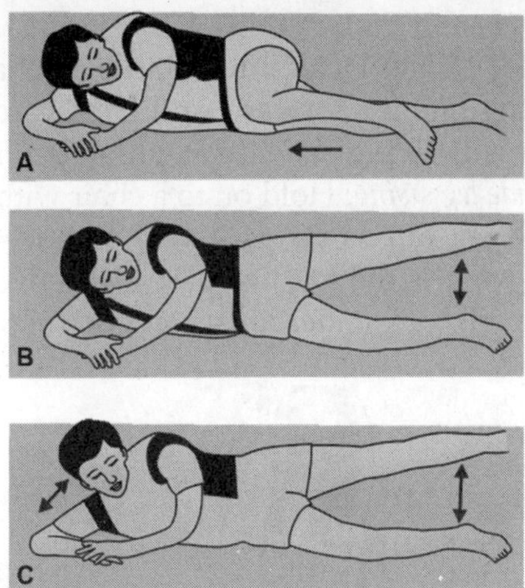

Figs 4.16A to C: Exercises lying on side: (A) Knee and hip flexion, and, (B, C) side leg raising

- *Feet together, knees apart:* Keep the ankles together and move the knees apart, then relax (Fig. 4.17B).

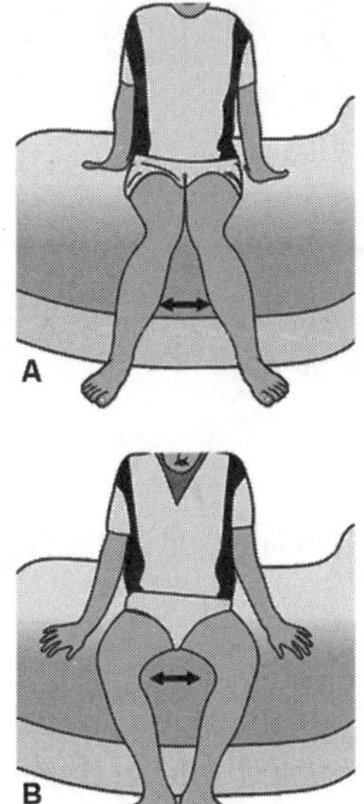

Figs 4.17A and B: Exercises while sitting: (A) Knees together, feet apart, and (B) Feet together, knees apart

Exercises in Standing Posture (Figs 4.18A and B)

- *Standing leg swing:* Hold into a table or chair with one hand, swing one leg forward and backward. Try to get the backwards swing as wide as possible (Fig. 4.18A).
- *Standing side leg swing:* Hold on to a chair with both hands. Swing bad leg out as far as it will go and then in. The outward swing is the hardest part and the leg should be allowed to fall back under muscular control (Fig. 4.18B).

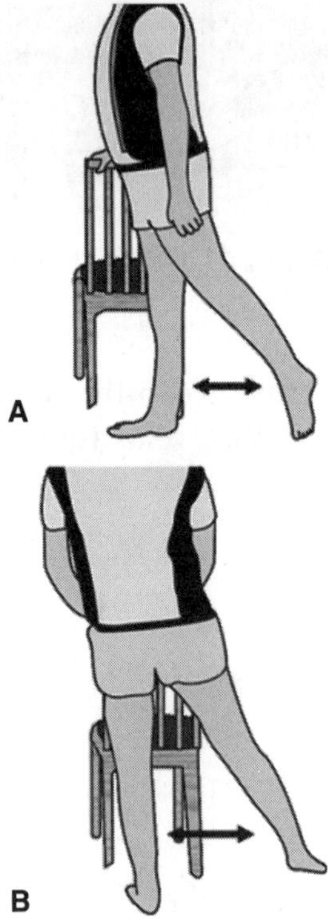

Figs 4.18A and B: (A) Standing swing, and (B) Standing side leg swing

Osteoarthritis of the Small Joints

Osteoarthritis may affect the peripheral joints of the hand and foot. It may cause ankylosis at an increased rate in these joints (Figs 4.19 and 4.20).

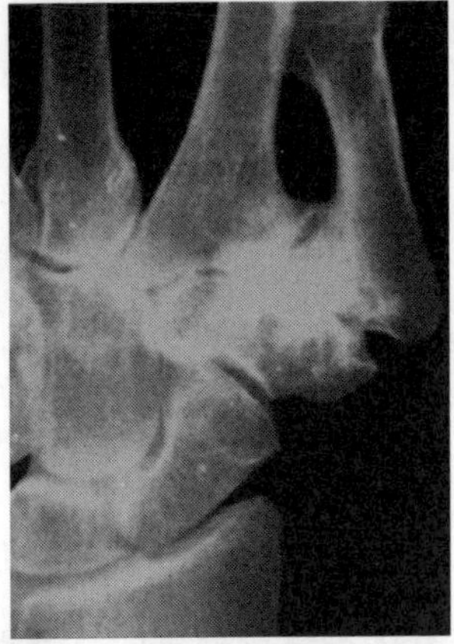

Fig. 4.19: Radiograph showing carpometacarpal joint of the thumb: Loss of joint space and sclerosis

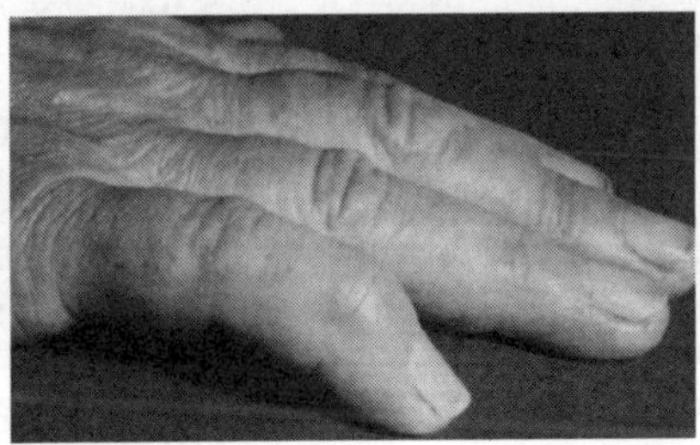

Fig. 4.20: Clinical photograph of OA hand

Remember in osteoarthritis of other joints

- Heberden's node—osteophytes around distal interphalangeal joints of the hand.
- Bouchard's node—osteophytes along proximal interphalangeal joints (Fig. 4.20).
- Mucinous cysts—cysts containing degenerative myxomatous fibrous tissue at the distal or proximal interphalangeal joints.
- Bunion is a combination of osteoarthritis and valgus angulation of the first metatarsophalangeal joint of foot.
- Erosive osteoarthritis: It is a hereditary severe osteoarthritis involving distal and proximal interphalangeal joints. Joint deformities and ankylosis result more often.

- Osteoarthritis of the first carpometacarpal joint of the thumb—seen in women more than 50 years (Fig. 4.20). They complain of pain and loss of grip.
- Osteoarthritis of the wrist—seen in Kienbock's disease, trauma, gout, nonunion scaphoid, etc.
- Osteoarthritis of the acromioclavicular joint—this is quite common.
- Osteoarthritis of the ankle joint though not as common as OA knee but is increasingly being seen of late and leads to troublesome pain and limp (Fig. 4.21).
- Osteoarthritis of the shoulder joint is rare and is not as common as OA hip joint (Fig. 4.22).

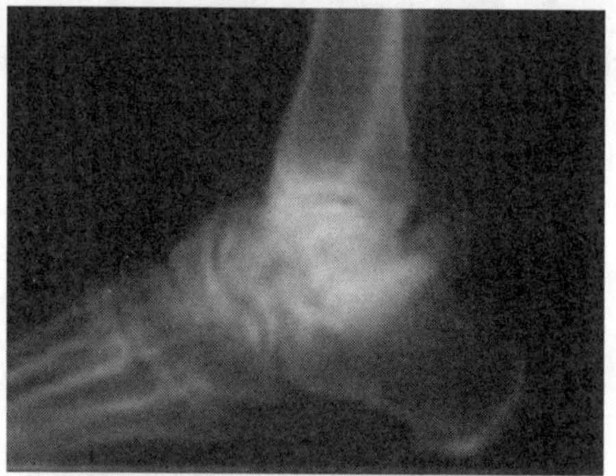

Fig. 4.21: Radiograph showing OA ankle

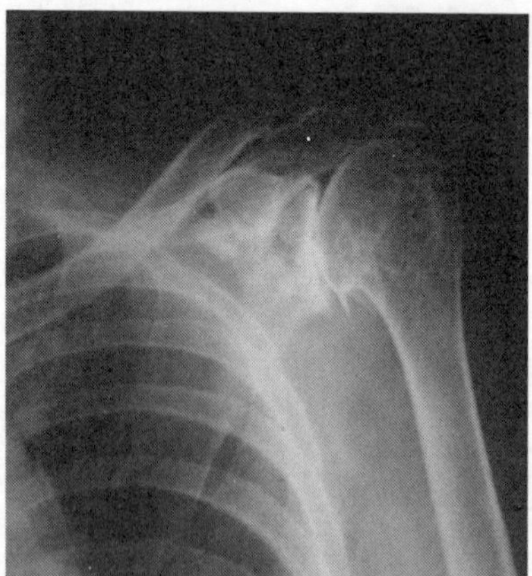

Fig. 4.22: Radiograph showing OA shoulder

BIBLIOGRAPHY

1. Cach JE. Cash's Textbook of Orthopedics and Rheumatology for Physiotherapists, Downe, DA (Ed). London, Boston, Faber and Faber, 1984.
2. Cooper NJ, Mageford M, et al. Secondary Health Service Care and second line drugs, costs of early inflammatory in Nortflok, UK. J Rheumatoid 2000:27:2115–22.
3. Goldberg VM. Surgery for rheumatoid disease: Part 2: Early management of the rheumatoid joint. In American Academy of Orthopedic Surgeons. Instructional Course Lectures. Vol. 33, St Louis, 1984, The CV Mosby Co.
4. Hill DF, Holbrook WP. Prevention and treatment of deformities in rheumatoid arthritis. JAMA 1950; 142:718.
5. Imaging in rheumatology. Medicine International 75, 3100.
6. Neustadt DH. HLA antigens in rheumatic diseases. Orthop Rev 1977; 6:19.

Index